GLOBAL SPREAD OF THE AVIAN FLU: ISSUES AND ACTIONS

GLOBAL SPREAD OF THE AVIAN FLU: ISSUES AND ACTIONS

MARILYN R. BETHE
EDITOR

Novinka Books
An imprint of Nova Science Publishers, Inc.
New York

For permission to use material from this book please contact us:
Telephone 631-231-7269; Fax 631-231-8175
Web Site: http://www.novapublishers.com

Library of Congress Cataloging-in-Publication Data:
Global spread of the avian flu : issues and actions / Marilyn R. Bethe, editor.
p. ; cm.
Includes bibliographical references and index.
ISBN 1-60021-011-2
1. Avian influenza--Prevention. 2. Avian influenza A virus. 3. Zoonoses--Prevention. I. Bethe, Marilyn R.
[DNLM: 1. Influenza in Birds--epidemiology. 2. Disease Outbreaks--prevention & control. 3. Influenza A Virus, H5N1 Subtype--pathogenicity. 4. Influenza in Birds--transmission. 5. Influenza, Human--prevention & control. SF 995.6.I6 G562 2006]
RA644.I6G56 2006
614.5'18--dc22 2006002031

Published by Nova Science Publishers, Inc. ✣ New York

CONTENTS

PREFACE

Avian influenza, or "bird flu", is a contagious disease of animals caused by viruses that normally infect only birds and, less commonly, pigs. Avian influenza viruses are highly species-specific, but have, on rare occasions, crossed the species barrier to infect humans. In domestic poultry, infection with avian influenza viruses causes two main forms of disease, distinguished by low and high extremes of virulence. The so-called "low pathogenic" form commonly causes only mild symptoms (ruffled feathers, a drop in egg production) and may easily go undetected. The highly pathogenic form is far more dramatic. It spreads very rapidly through poultry flocks, causes disease affecting multiple internal organs, and has a mortality that can approach 100%, often within 48 hours.

A pandemic can start when three conditions have been met: a new influenza virus subtype emerges; it infects humans, causing serious illness; and it spreads easily and sustainably among humans. The H5N1 virus amply meets the first two conditions: it is a new virus for humans (H5N1 viruses have never circulated widely among people), and it has infected more than 100 humans, killing over half of them. No one will have immunity should an H5N1-like pandemic virus emerge.

All prerequisites for the start of a pandemic have therefore been met save one: the establishment of efficient and sustained human-to-human transmission of the virus. The risk that the H5N1 virus will acquire this ability will persist as long as opportunities for human infections occur. These opportunities, in turn, will persist as long as the virus continues to circulate in birds, and this situation could endure for some years to come.

In: Global Spread of the Avian Flu… ISBN 1-60021-011-2
Editors: M.R. Bethe, pp. 1-58

Chapter 1

U.S. AND INTERNATIONAL RESPONSES TO THE GLOBAL SPREAD OF AVIAN FLU *

Tiaji Salaam-Blyther and Emma Chanlett-Avery

SUMMARY

One strain of avian influenza currently identified in Asia and Europe is known as Influenza A/H5N1. Although it is a bird flu, it has infected a relatively small number of people — killing around 50% of those infected. Scientists are unsure if H5N1 will cause the next influenza pandemic, but there is general consensus that one is overdue. Flu pandemics have occurred cyclically, roughly between every 30 and 50 years. Since 1997, when the first human contracted H5N1 in Hong Kong, the virus has resurfaced and spread to more than a dozen countries in Asia and Europe — infecting more than 140 people and killing approximately half. Britain and Taiwan both reported avian flu cases of H5N1 in 2005. In the latter cases, the infected birds were identified as imports, and died in quarantine.

A global influenza pandemic could have a number of consequences. Global competition for existing vaccines and treatments could ensue. Some governments might restrict the export of vaccines or other supplies in order to treat their own population. Some countries might face a shortage of vaccines, antiviral medication, or other

* Excerpted from CRS Report RL33219, dated January 9, 2006.

medical equipment, because of limited global supply. Hospitality and airline industries, and international trade could be negatively impacted. If global travel and trade were to suddenly drop, there could be productivity losses and service disruptions. Essential workers might become ill or stay home out of fear of contracting the virus. Such workers could include law enforcement, medical personnel, mass transit drivers and engineers, and other crucial emergency personnel.

For FY2006, Congress has provided $25 million for global initiatives to prepare for pandemic influenza through Foreign Operations appropriations; directed $33.5 million to global disease detection through Labor, HHS, and Education appropriations; and reserved for international avian flu efforts a portion of $3.8 billion through Defense appropriations.

Bills introduced in the 109th Congress would increase U.S. resources allocated to the global fight against avian flu; develop a "Pandemic Fund" to augment ongoing U.S. and international avian flu and pandemic preparedness initiatives; increase funding for preventing the spread among animals of the H5N1 virus; and strengthen surveillance capacity within affected countries.

This chapter provides an up-to-date account of global H5N1-related human infections and deaths, outline U.S. government and international responses to the global spread of H5N1, discuss situations in various countries affected by H5N1, and present some foreign policy issues for Congress.

BACKGROUND

Bird (or avian) flu outbreaks have occurred at various times around the world.[1] One strain of avian influenza currently spreading across Asia and Europe is known as Influenza A/H5N1. Although it is a bird flu, it has also infected a relatively small number of people — killing around 50% of those infected. Until 1997, there were no known cases of humans contracting avian influenza. However, that year, 18 people in Hong Kong contracted the virus; of those 6 died. To stop its spread, 1.5 million birds were killed. Since 2003, scientists have closely monitored resurgent H5N1 outbreaks, which have infected chickens and ducks in a growing number of countries. The World Health Organization is particularly alarmed about the rapid spread of H5N1 in part, because this strain of bird flu has demonstrated the ability to cause high mortality rates among humans.

According to WHO, the hallmarks of a pandemic are: 1) a novel influenza virus strain emerges; 2) the strain causes human disease; and 3) person-to-person transmission is sustained. The pandemic steps usually occur in six phases. Table 1 shows the phases of an influenza pandemic, as described by WHO. The WHO considers the recent H5N1 outbreak to be in phase three pandemic alert phase, which means a virus new to humans is causing infections, but does not spread easily from one person to another.[2]

Since H5N1 is a bird flu, and has not commonly infected people, humans have no immunity against it. If H5N1 were to become transmissible among humans, an "influenza pandemic" (worldwide disease outbreak) could begin, potentially causing millions of deaths. Skeptics argue that predictions that H5N1 might cause a global pandemic are exaggerated, because if the virus were able to become efficiently transmissible among people it would have already transformed.

Still a growing number of health experts underscore that it is critical for governments to prepare for some form of an influenza pandemic, as the world is overdue for one. During the influenza pandemic of 1918-1919 (Spanish flu), estimates are that between 20 and 50 million people died, and between 200 million and 1 billion were infected around the world. If an influenza pandemic were to occur on the same scale as the Spanish flu, some estimate that between 30 million and 384 million people could die around the world,[3] of which 1.9 million deaths could occur in the United States.[4]

Global Prevalence

Since 1997, when the first human contracted H5N1 in Hong Kong, the virus has resurfaced and spread to birds in fifteen countries, ten in Asia and five in Europe.[5] In 2004, nine Asian countries reported H5N1 poultry outbreaks: Cambodia, China, Indonesia, Japan, Laos, Malaysia, Republic of Korea, Thailand, and Vietnam. By August 2005, birds in Mongolia had become infected with the virus. Two months later, in October, domestic birds in Russia and Kazakhstan had contracted H5N1 reportedly through contact with wild waterfowl at shared water sources. By late October 2005, H5N1 had spread progressively westward to affect six other regions in Russia, and had infected bird populations in Romania, Croatia, and Turkey. Although human infection has not been reported outside Asia, health officials are wary about infection among migratory birds, as the birds are currently acting as vectors of the virus. Also, infection can potentially be controlled among domestic birds, but not among wild ones. The chart below shows the latest number of confirmed human H5N1 cases as reported by WHO as of December 30, 2005[6]. The map in the Annex (Chart 1) illustrates the human H5N1 cases.

Table 1. Human Cases of Avian Influenza A/H5N1

Indonesia		Vietnam		Thailand		Cambodia		China		Turkey	
Cases	Deaths	Cases	Deaths	Cases	Deaths	Cases	Deaths	Cases	Deaths	Cases	Deaths
16	11	93	42	22	14	4	4	7	3	4	2
Total Cases = 146; Total Deaths = 76											

CONGRESSIONAL RESPONSE

Congress provided $25 million to support ongoing U.S. efforts to prevent and contain the spread of H5N1 through P.L. 109-13, *FY2005 Emergency Supplemental Appropriations*. The act, which passed in May 2005, also provided funds for domestic pandemic preparedness.[7] Additionally, the act directed U.S. agencies to develop a coordinated response to the global spread of H5N1. Congress provided the funds to U.S. Agency for International Development (USAID). Pursuant to the statute, USAID transferred $15 million of the $25 million appropriation to CDC.

The conference report for P.L. 109-102, *FY2006 Foreign Operations Appropriations,* urges the United States Executive Director to the World Bank to use the voice and vote of the United States to increase support for using International Development Association (IDA) funds to help eligible countries prepare for and combat a potential avian influenza epidemic. Particularly, the report points out that funds could be used in Asia for programs to increase surveillance capacity, compensate small-scale farmers for timely reports of bird die-offs, modernize animal husbandry practices, and upgrade infectious disease infrastructure. The report also underscores that the $25 million provided in P.L. 109-13 is the first step in a multi-year effort to contain, prevent, and prepare for the spread of avian influenza.

H.Rept. 109-337 for H.R. 3010, *FY2006 Labor, HHS, and Education Appropriations*, includes $63.58 million for the Public Health and Social Services Emergency Fund (PHSSEF) to enhance federal, state, and local preparedness to counter potential biological, disease, chemical, and radiological threats to civilian populations. Additionally, $33.5 million is directed to global disease detection. The bill does not include funds to support the President's FY2006 $7.1 billion emergency request for avian flu and pandemic influenza preparedness. Instead, appropriators provided additional funds through FY2006 Defense Appropriations. The *FY2006 Defense, Disaster Assistance, and Avian Flu Preparedness Appropriations* conference report, H.Rept. 109-359, reserves a portion of the $3.8 billion directed to avian flu activities for international avian flu efforts.[8] The Senate passed the House version after removing a controversial provision related to oil drilling in Alaska. H.R. 3010 and H.R. 2863 were presented to the President on December 28, 2005.

Table 3 reflects FY2006 appropriations that include funding for global avian flu activities.

Press reports quote a number of Members expressing concern about funding the President's $7.1 billion avian flu and pandemic preparedness request. The Chairman of the House Energy and Commerce Committee, Joe Barton, reportedly stated that he would not support funding for the bill if the President did not provide offsets for avian flu and pandemic preparedness spending.[9] Others proposed that Congress spread out funding the request over a few years.

Some congressional Members argued that the Administration has allocated insufficient resources to the global fight against H5N1 and pandemic planning. Of the $7.1 billion requested, approximately $388 million would be reserved for global efforts. A number of Members have introduced legislation to increase U.S. resources allocated to the global fight against avian flu. Some bills, such as H.R. 4062,

Pandemic Preparedness and Responsibility Act and its Senate companion, S. 1821, propose developing a "Pandemic Fund"to augment ongoing U.S. and international avian flu and pandemic preparedness initiatives. Other bills, such as H.R. 4476,

Global Network for Avian Influenza Surveillance Act, and its Senate companion, S. 1912, advocate greater support for initiatives that prevent the spread of H5N1 among animals. A number of bills, such as H.R. 3369, *Attacking Viral Influenza Across Nations Act*, and its Senate companion, S. 969, suggest the U.S. strengthen surveillance capacity within affected countries. Bills, such as H.R. 813, *Flu Protection Act*, and its Senate companion, S. 375, aim to boost influenza vaccine supply. Additionally, other legislation, such as H.R. 4245, *Influenza Preparedness and Prevention Act* encourage greater international cooperation.

Some Members of Congress have also expressed support for greater spending on global initiatives during congressional hearings. For example, during the House International Relations Committee hearing on pandemic flu in December 2005, Chairman Henry Hyde questioned whether the amount the President requested for international pandemic flu preparedness was sufficient. A number of other committees have also held hearings on avian flu and pandemic preparedness, including the Senate Foreign Relations and Appropriations Committees, House Agriculture Committee and a joint hearing by the House Homeland Security and Armed Services Committees.

U.S. Executive Branch Response

On November 1, 2005, the President released the National Strategy for Pandemic Influenza. One day later, on November 2, 2005, the Administration released the U.S. Department of Health and Human Services (HHS) Influenza Plan. The HHS plan provided a detailed explanation of how the national strategy would be implemented. Some were disappointed by the relatively small proportion of funds reserved for international efforts. It has been argued that greater investment in pandemic influenza preparedness abroad could enhance domestic pandemic preparedness efforts. Of the $7.1 billion requested, approximately $388 million is reserved for global initiatives. Of the $388 million, $200 million is made available for HHS to bolster international surveillance capacity; $131.5 million for USAID to implement avian influenza containment efforts globally; an additional $18.5 million for the State Department for avian flu and pandemic preparedness activities in diplomatic arenas, $20 million for the potential evacuation of U.S. government personnel and their dependents in the event of a pandemic; and $18.3 million for the Department of Agriculture to provide technical assistance in international animal surveillance.[10] Table 2 summarizes the FY2006 emergency request.

HHS (and its relevant agencies), USAID, the Department of Agriculture, and the Department of Defense are the key U.S. departments and agency involved in containing the global spread of H5N1 and preparing for pandemic influenza. The Department of State plays a complementary role by raising the issue in diplomatic arenas. The unique role that each agency plays is described in order of presence on the ground.

Prior to 2005 — when Congress provided $25 million for preventing the global spread of avian influenza and preparing for pandemic influenza — U.S. agencies had been enhancing laboratory capabilities, training health care providers, strengthening surveillance systems, and developing influenza pandemic plans. Through the FY2005 emergency appropriations, Congress directed U.S. agencies to revisit international influenza initiatives and ensure that there was a coordinated response to the global spread of H5N1. USAID and HHS (including its relevant agencies) undertook country planning visits to Vietnam, Cambodia, and Laos. After the trip, the team outlined in a report[11] a number of factors that have complicated efforts to contain the spread of H5N1 in Vietnam, Cambodia, and Laos, which included:

- Between 70% and 80% of poultry in the three countries are raised in small backyard farms, hindering national governments' ability to ensure health standards.
- Between 50% and 80% of poultry die from other avian infections, complicating efforts to identify unusual die-offs, and limiting farmers' likelihood of reporting bird deaths to authorities.
- Although culling is an essential element of controlling the spread of H5N1, poorer countries can not afford to systematically compensate farmers for lost stock, which also increases reluctance to report signs of infection.
- Wild birds and domesticated ducks are H5N1 reservoirs.
- Low levels of awareness exist among local farmers.
- There is little pandemic preparedness activity in the countries toured.
- The capacity to monitor and respond effectively to animal outbreaks is limited. Veterinary services are inadequate to deal with the scope, severity, and rapid spread of H5N1 epidemics, which has resulted in the disease becoming increasingly endemic among animal populations in the region. The lack of human resources for disease surveillance, diagnostics, and response also severely limits the capacity of human health systems, and continued human infections of avian influenza threaten to overburden already fragile public health infrastructures.

The report also included an action plan, which outlined the activities that each agency would implement. The agency-specific strategies are briefly described below. Table 4 provides a country-specific illustration of Department of Health and Human Services (HHS) and USAID spending for the FY2005 Emergency Supplemental Appropriations.

U.S. Department of Health and Human Services (HHS)

CDC is the key agency at HHS responsible for implementing U.S. anti-influenza activities around the world. The Coordinating Center for Infectious

Diseases and the Field Epidemiology Training Program — a CDC-sponsored activity — are also critical components of HHS global pandemic preparedness initiatives. Activities with foreign governments or populations include pandemic preparedness and planning; training in avian influenza surveillance; laboratory safety and skills instruction; epidemiology training; developing and training rapid response teams; stockpiling support; and deployment of expert disease control teams.

It is not possible to disaggregate H5N1-specific funding, because H5N1, seasonal flu, and pandemic preparedness initiatives are interlocked. A significant part of H5N1 and pandemic influenza planning is funded through the Global Disease Detection (GDD) Initiative at CDC. GDD aims to recognize infectious disease outbreaks faster, improve the ability to control and prevent outbreaks, and detect emerging microbial threats. CDC estimates that in FY2004, it spent approximately $5 million on activities related to international influenza through both its Infectious Diseases Control and GDD programs. In FY2005, CDC spent approximately $6 million through these activities, in addition to the $15 million emergency appropriations. In 2005, CDC expanded its GDD activities by creating new sites, improving early warning systems, researching new viral strains, and supporting international organizations. Congress provided $21.4 million for GDD in FY2005.The HHS FY2006 budget request suggests increasing GDD funding by $12.1 million to $33.5 million, of which a portion would be used for international bird flu initiatives.[12] H. Rept.109-337, *FY2006 Labor, HHS, and Education Appropriations* directed $33.5 million to GDD.

U.S. Agency for International Development (USAID)

USAID coordinates its global H5N1 and influenza response with other U.S. agencies. It also works closely with the WHO, the Food and Agriculture Organization of the United Nations (FAO), and other international governments and organizations to support national influenza and H5N1 prevention efforts. To date, the agency has spent $13.7 million on avian influenza prevention and containment ($10 million of which was funded through the FY2005 emergency appropriations).[13] Specifically, the agency has:

- dedicated $7.5 million to Cambodia, China, Indonesia, Laos, and Vietnam for strengthening disease surveillance, laboratory diagnosis, and rapid containment of animal outbreaks;

- provided $2.85 million for communication campaigns in Laos, Cambodia, Vietnam, and Indonesia aimed at reducing animal handling practices that place humans at risk;
- committed over $1.6 million to enhance national planning efforts, strengthen avian influenza control and outbreak response, and augment human disease surveillance systems and laboratories;
- granted WHO $300,000 for international coordination efforts and for improving disease control and surveillance measures;
- provided WHO an additional$250,000 for personal protective equipment (PPE) used in handling and disposing of infected poultry; and
- distributed some 10,000 sets of PPEs, which include manual sprayers to assist in decontaminating hospital rooms and equipment, Tyvek suits (protective coveralls used in hazardous situations), gloves, boots, masks, and eye protection in Cambodia, Thailand, Laos, Vietnam, and Indonesia.

The Administration's FY2006 emergency supplemental request allocates $131.5 million to USAID for avian flu and pandemic preparedness initiatives abroad. The funds would be used to pre-position supplies and equipment that prevent and control the spread of avian influenza; launch awareness raising campaigns; and accelerate international planning and preparedness. The request proposes that $2 million of the USAID funds be reserved for initiatives in Russia and Eastern Europe.

Department of State

On September 14, 2005, President Bush announced the International Partnership on Avian and Pandemic Influenza (IPAPI) at the U.N. General Assembly High-Level Plenary Session. IPAPI seeks to generate and coordinate political momentum and action for addressing the threats of avian and pandemic influenza based on a set of core principles. The principles are focused on enhancing preparedness, prevention, response, and containment activities (see Table 5). The Partnership brings key nations and international organizations together to improve global readiness by:

- elevating the issue of avian and pandemic influenza preparedness to the national level;
- coordinating efforts among donor and affected nations;

- mobilizing and leveraging resources;
- increasing transparency in disease reporting and surveillance; and
- building capacity to identify, contain, and respond to pandemic influenza.

The State Department works closely with regional organizations, including the Association of Southeast Asian Nations (ASEAN) and the Asia Pacific Economic Cooperation (APEC) forum, to address avian influenza and the threat of an influenza pandemic. The work includes efforts to encourage comprehensive national pandemic preparedness plans that address the multi-sectoral impacts of an influenza pandemic.[14]

In the FY2006 supplemental request, the President proposed that the State Department receive $38.5 million in FY2006 for international response coordination; diplomatic outreach; exchanges of U.S. and foreign medical personnel; and for avian and pandemic influenza health support and protection of U.S. government employees and families at U.S. missions overseas. About $20 million of those funds would be reserved for the potential evacuation of U.S. government personnel and dependents from overseas missions.

Department of Agriculture (USDA)

U.S. Department of Agriculture (and its related agencies)works closely with other U.S. agencies on the ground, as well as other international organizations to help nations take steps to address and control the spread of avian influenza. Dr. Ron DeHaven, Administrator, Animal and Plant Health Inspection Service (APHIS) of USDA stated that addressing avian flu at its source — in affected poultry abroad —and participating in international eradication efforts provide the best opportunity to reduce or eliminate the risk of an H5N1 pandemic.[15] In that view, USDA and other analysts consider the department's efforts a critical element in the global fight against the spread of H5N1.

Through $4 million in FY2003 emergency funding, APHIS launched an outreach campaign called "Biosecurity for the Birds," which provides poultry farmers with the latest information on biosecurity to prevent the spread of avian infections on farms. USDA is translating the brochures for use in southeast Asia.

Additionally, in the FY2006 emergency supplemental, the President requests $91.3 million for USDA, of which $18.3 million is reserved for international initiatives. The would be allocated as follows:

- $8.0 million for wildlife, poultry and swine surveillance and diagnostics;
- $1.75 million for biosecurity enhancement through education and information;
- $1.05 million for technical assistance through training and avian movement control;
- $3.8 million for training and education related to industry changes and food safety planning;
- $1.05 million for training and education regarding poultry destruction and disposal methods;
- $0.6 million for testing and evaluation of vaccine formulations; and
- $2.1 million for in country expertise for longer term assistance.

Department of Defense (DOD)

The Department of Defense Global Emerging Infections System (GEIS) delivers health care to American armed forces around the globe.[16] GEIS has a network of overseas medical research laboratories that track, prevent, and treat infectious diseases around the world. The objective is to protect the U.S. military and strengthen its ability to address the challenges related to a potential pandemic influenza, including compromised military force health and readiness. GEIS is also a critical partner in the WHO's Global Outbreak Alert and Response Network (GOARN) (described below). Key DoD-GEIS activities to combat the spread of H5N1 and prepare for an influenza pandemic have included:

- providing a DoD staff veterinarian to serve as a member of the WHO GOARN Team in Laos, and to conduct training workshops in detecting and diagnosing avian flu cases;
- placing a U.S. Navy microbiologist at the Institute Pasteur in Ho Chi Minh City, Vietnam, to hold training sessions on rapid diagnostic test methodology;
- monitoring and preventing infectious disease emergence in southeast Asia through its Armed Forces Research Institute of Medical Sciences (AFRIMS).[17]

The Naval Medical Research Unit-2 (NAMRU-2) is another critical part of DoD's effort to prevent H5N1 from becoming a human pandemic and prepare for an influenza pandemic. NAMRU-2 supports the GEIS mission through four programs: emerging diseases, enteric diseases, parasitic diseases, and virology. NAMRU-2 is an overseas research laboratory based in Jakarta, Indonesia with related activities in Southeast Asia and the Pacific Islands. NAMRU-2 also supports a satellite laboratory in Phnom Penh, Cambodia, in collaboration with the Cambodian National Institute of Public Health. Key activities include:

- bolstering local, national, and regional diagnostic and epidemiological capacity;
- assisting in the development of new surveillance strategies, such as the novel syndromic surveillance initiative Early Warning Outbreak Recognition System (EWORS);
- implementing a comprehensive influenza surveillance project in Indonesia, which provides prevalence data and temporal, genotype data of circulating strains;
- collaborating with CDC in its FY2005 and FY2006 global influenza activities; and
- facilitating the transformation of outbreak response structures into more effective, multidisciplinary, centrally directed ones.[18]

The FY2006 emergency supplemental request would reserve $10 million of the $130 million allocated to the Department of Defense for procuring protective equipment; laboratory diagnostic equipment; portable field assay testing equipment; and surveillance and communication equipment.

INTERNATIONAL RESPONSE[19]

Overview of the Role of the World Health Organization

The World Health Organization, established in 1948, is the U.N. system's authority on international public health issues. It assists governments to improve national health services and establish worldwide standards for foods, chemicals, and biological and pharmaceutical products. WHO concentrates on preventive rather than curative programs, including efforts to eradicate endemic and other widespread diseases, stabilize population growth, and improve nutrition, sanitation, and maternal and child care. WHO works through contracts with other agencies and private voluntary organizations. The United States has been a member of WHO since its inception.

WHO is a central actor in the global response to the outbreak of H5N1 avian influenza. As in the case of SARS in 2003, WHO seeks to mitigate the risks avian influenza and infectious diseases pose to international public health, and to assure the availability of appropriate containment mechanisms, particularly since global travel has become the primary means of spreading disease around the world. With the exception of SARS and HIV/AIDS, H5N1 is viewed as the most serious challenge the WHO has faced in the last few decades.

Who's Global Health Security

The Epidemic and Pandemic Alert and Response system is a critical part of WHO's global health security plan. Key aspects of the program include:

- **The Alert and Response Operations**: systematically track the development of diseases, share and disseminate information, and coordinate rapid outbreak response and logistics.
- **The Global Outbreak Alert and Response Network (GOARN):** provides an operational framework and aims to create a standardized international outbreak response system through 112 institutions and networks of people and technical resources.[20]
- **The Global Public Health Intelligence Network (GPHIN)**: tracks Internet communications through a customized search engine, which effectively picked up telecommunicated alerts in China during the SARS outbreak. WHO also uses the system to clarify or refute information that may create disruption or panic.

Who Global Influenza Preparedness Plan[21]

In September 2005, U.N. Secretary-General Kofi Annan appointed Dr. David Nabarro as the Senior U.N. System Coordinator for Human and Avian influenza. Dr. Nabarro, seconded from the WHO, is responsible for coordinating the avian influenza containment efforts of the various U.N. agencies. Dr. Nabarro is also tasked with encouraging global support and implementation of the WHO Global Influenza Preparedness Plan. The plan outlines WHO goals and actions, as well as recommended actions for individual nations, at each pandemic phase (see Table 1). The plan contains an annex of recommendations to nations for "non-pharmaceutical public health interventions," such as isolation, quarantine and travel restrictions. The annex stresses the use of voluntary rather than compulsory measures. Additionally, it stresses that nations implement infection-specific responses, noting the lack of demonstrated utility of certain practices. For example, certain SARS control measures, such as temperature screening at airports, would not be expected to effectively control influenza spread.[22]

WHO has requested \$150 million to establish a global stockpile of influenza vaccines and treatments. WHO officials underscore that wealthy and poor countries must develop pandemic preparedness plans collectively to reduce national and international viral transmission. The organization envisions using the stockpile to arrest a potential pandemic by containing the virus at the first sign of an outbreak. In the event of an outbreak, WHO asserts that a pandemic could potentially be averted if antiviral drugs were quickly distributed in a poor country without access to them.[23] To date, countries have pledged between \$20 million and \$30 million to fund the stockpile. Roche, the patent holder of Tamiflu, announced that it would donate three million courses of the drug to WHO[24]. The company estimates that the three million courses would be ready before mid-2006.

Similarly, the U.N. General Assembly has established an emergency fund —Central Emergency Response Fund (CERF) — to provide quick initial funding during the early stages of emergencies and to minimize extra costs related to funding delays. The U.N. aims to have a \$500 million revolving budget that could be used within three to four days of the start of an emergency. To date, the United Nations has received more than \$200 million for the fund, which will be launched in mid-January and should be operational by March.[25]

Role of other International Health Organizations

The U.N. Food and Agriculture Organization coordinates global surveillance and response activities for animal influenza strains with pandemic potential, such as H5N1.[26] To accomplish its mission, FAO works closely with the World Organization for Animal Health, known by its French acronym, OIE.[27] Rapid detection of avian influenza outbreaks is key to controlling the disease both in poultry and in people, and is therefore key to preventing and controlling a potential influenza pandemic. FAO, OIE, and WHO work closely to prevent and respond to the threat of an avian influenza pandemic. FAO has spent $7.5 million on H5N1 initiatives since 2004. USAID is granting the UN organization $6 million, and the German government has pledged $20 million for 2005 and 2006 activities.[28] FAO is requesting an additional $175 million from the international community, due to the rapid global spread of H5N1.

The World Bank provides low-interest loans to countries heavily affected by H5N1. Additionally, the Bank coordinates efforts between countries, and encourages them to develop pandemic plans that connect sectors, such as health and rural development. In September 2005, representatives from the WHO, FAO, OIE and the World Bank met with health experts from the United Nations, European Commission and H5N1-affected countries to discuss the global spread of H5N1, to emphasize the importance of pandemic planning, and to prepare a coordinated response. On November 4, 2005, the World Bank announced that it would provide $500 million in loans to poor southeast Asian countries that are struggling to combat avian influenza. The funds will be used to supplement government resources, strengthen veterinary systems, and assist in culling and animal vaccination programs.[29] Although the World Bank has agreed to provide $500 million in loans to affected countries, the Bank estimates that $1 billion could be needed over the next three years.[30] The $1 billion does not include the cost of financing human or animal vaccine development, purchasing antiviral medicine, or compensating farmers for loss of income.

The WHO, FAO, OIE, and the World Bank co-sponsored a meeting on avian influenza and human pandemic influenza on November 7-9, 2005, in Geneva, Switzerland, to develop an integrated global plan and to focus on funding initiatives.[31] Participants agreed to a six-point global plan which called for:

- Controlling the virus at its source in birds;
- Strengthening surveillance, early detection, rapid response systems, and laboratory capacity;
- Training national staff in investigating animal and human cases, and planning and testing rapid containment activities;
- Building and testing national pandemic preparedness plans, conducting a global pandemic response exercise, and enhancing health systems;
- Developing integrated country plans that encompass all sectors; and
- Ensuring factual and transparent communications.[32]

International Health Regulations

An outbreak of infectious diseases raises many public health questions including the application of international law, particularly as it affects three main areas —International Health Regulations (IHR); public health measures and civil and political rights; and principles of state responsibility.[33] This section will focus on the IHR because of its relevance to WHO.

On May 23, 2005, the World Health Assembly revised the IHR, adding novel influenza strains (those with pandemic potential) and SARS to the list of "notifiable diseases" that WHO urges countries to report. In addition, the revised IHR include a provision requiring notification of "events of international concern." This mechanism could strengthen WHO's ability to address emerging diseases, because it requires member States to report unusual health events whether or not they are attributable to a known pathogen. The updated IHR also include expanded requirements for disease surveillance and control activities at points of international travel (airports, border crossings, etc.), and urge developed countries to assist developing countries to gain the capacities needed to meet the new disease control guidelines.[34]

The revised IHR are to replace the existing IHR (adopted in 1969) on June 15, 2007, when the revised regulations come into force. Considered an international legal instrument, the revised IHR will be binding on all WHO member States who have not stated a reservation or rejected them altogether, and on non-member States that have notified the Director-General of WHO that they agree to be bound by the revised IHR.[35] Between now and June 2007, WHO and Member States may take concrete steps towards implementation of the revised IHR and to improve their capacity to respond to international health risks and emergencies.[36] The revised IHR do not include an enforcement mechanism. However, for states to respond appropriately and avoid potentially harmful consequences, much of the encouragement to comply will likely come from international pressure, as the SARS outbreak demonstrated.

AFFECTED COUNTRIES' RESPONSE

Degree and sophistication of preparation for avian influenza vary widely among the affected countries. The more affluent governments have undertaken more extensive measures as well as committed national resources to hedge against the risk of a pandemic. Japan and Taiwan have reportedly both accumulated stockpiles of Tamiflu and are preparing to manufacture their own supply. Singapore has reportedly stockpiled antivirals for 10% of its population, enhanced surveillance, and put a detailed contingency plan in place. WHO officials praised an exercise run by South Korea which simulated how the government would respond to an outbreak.[37] On the other hand, the closed governments of Burma (Myanmar) and North Korea offer little reliable information about the presence of bird flu within their borders. Although both Yangon and Pyongyang have provided limited cooperation with the FAO, their officially rosy outlooks are treated with skepticism by international health experts and could constitute a weak link in the event of a pandemic.

The profiles below focus on countries that have had cases of human infection. Although Russia has had no human cases to date, an analysis of H5N1 cases has been included, because H5N1 has spread to other parts of Europe from there. H5N1 cases in birds have been confirmed in Romania, Turkey, Kazakhstan, the Ukraine, and Croatia,[38] and Turkey confirmed two deaths from the virus in early 2006. Britain and Taiwan both reported cases of H5N1 in 2005. However, the incidences are not discussed here, as experts concluded that the imported birds were identified and died in quarantine, and are believed unlikely to have spread the disease.

Cambodia[39]

Between February and April 2005, four Cambodians were confirmed to have died from the H5N1 avian flu virus. All four victims lived in Kampot province, an area where 600 poultry reportedly had fallen ill and died in March 2005. Despite warnings, many villagers ate birds that had been sick because food is not plentiful. Health experts predict that more cases in Cambodia are likely, though the WHO has not reported any additional human cases. Health officials in Kampot are being taught how to identify symptoms of avian influenza and instructed to notify the provincial health department. In September 2005, more than 1,000 water birds were reportedly found dead in poultry farms in Batambang and several other provinces. None of the birds tested have been confirmed to have the H5N1 virus. The Cambodian government has cooperated fully with the WHO, but the government has limited capacity to contain outbreaks of the disease. Compared to Thailand, in Cambodia, poultry farms are smaller but more numerous, and many chickens roam freely, while transportation and communications links are far less developed; hence monitoring the nation's poultry stocks is more difficult. The U.S. government assessment team that visited Laos, Cambodia, and Vietnam in July 2005 reported that the U.S. government, FAO, and WHO have strong working relationships with relevant ministries in the Cambodian government, while over 200 international donors and NGOs operating in the country could play an effective role in mobilizing an effective response to an outbreak of avian flu. On October 12, 2005, U.S. Secretary of Health and Human Services Michael Leavitt, on a visit to Southeast Asia, signed a cooperation agreement with Cambodian officials pledging $1.8 million to Cambodia to help the country guard against the spread of H5N1.[40] United Nations experts estimated that Cambodia needs $18 million to develop programs to stem the spread of the virus. In December 2005, Germany announced that it would provide $3 million to the kingdom to help fight the disease.[41]

People's Republic of China, Including Hong Kong[42]

The November 2005 confirmation of the first human cases and deaths from H5N1 in China in 2005 renewed fears that the spread of H5N1 could accelerate within China.[43] The close proximity of millions of people, birds, and animals in southern China has made it a common breeding ground for deadly types of influenza viruses, including the H5N1 avian flu virus, that jump the species barrier to humans. Added to this, the PRC's poor public health infrastructure and the traditionally secretive, un-transparent policy approach of its communist government have made international health specialists particularly concerned about the PRC as a possible contributor to an H5N1 flu global pandemic. Health care specialists have cited the PRC government's early lack of cooperation during the outbreak of Severe Acute Respiratory Syndrome, or SARS — a previously unknown virus that surfaced in southern China in 2003 — as a principal cause for that virus' quick global spread before it was contained.[44] As of January 1, 2006, there have been 31 outbreaks of the H5N1 strain in Chinese poultry since late October 2005, heightening international health concerns.

Hong Kong in late 1997 is where the H5N1 avian flu virus for the first time was recorded as jumping directly from its traditional animal species to humans, infecting 18 people in Hong Kong and killing six. Although the Hong Kong government responded aggressively at that time, in three days exterminating its entire poultry population of 1.5 million birds, the 1997 outbreak marked the beginning of the cycle of H5N1 outbreaks that expanded on a much wider scale throughout Asia in late 2003 and early

2004. On January 27, 2004, a WHO official stated that a "staggering" number of birds, both migratory and domestic, were infected with the virus in at least ten Asian countries. That same day in 2004, the PRC became the tenth country to acknowledge ongoing outbreaks of avian flu within its borders. According to WHO, H5N1 is now considered endemic in parts of China. In addition to afflicting domestic poultry and migratory birds in isolated parts of China, H5N1 also has been documented in parts of China's pig population.[45]

The 2003 SARS experience appears to have made PRC leaders more sensitive to potential catastrophic health issues. Consequently, Beijing has been far more assertive in enacting measures to combat the H5N1 virus. But even with the positive steps that have been taken, PRC officials face enormous problems in implementation. The PRC Ministry of Health reports it has established 63 influenza monitoring labs throughout most of China[46] and has crafted and published an emergency plan for an influenza pandemic, including a four-color-coded notification system.[47] On November 21, 2005, PRC agricultural officials at a press conference further announced the adoption and immediate implementation of contingency regulations to combat the spread of the disease and to punish government officials that delay or obfuscate medical and scientific reports about the virus. The regulations include requirements that provincial and municipal level officials notify the central government within four hours after a new flu outbreak.

By November 2005, PRC officials confirmed that they had either destroyed or vaccinated millions of healthy domestic poultry and that they were planning to inoculate the entire Chinese poultry population, a massive effort which would include as many as 14 billion chickens, geese, and ducks.[48] As a logistical effort, the initiative faces daunting difficulties — first among them the sheer size of China's poultry population and the fact that the poultry industry is widely scattered, including millions of rural households with a dozen or fewer chickens that roam free. Second, according to medical experts, the poultry vaccine to be fully effective must be given in two separate doses about a month apart, meaning the entire undertaking has to be performed twice for a single inoculation to be effective.[49] In addition, some health officials have expressed concern that such a broad campaign could backfire and actually contribute to spreading the disease further. Potential problems include the use of unlicensed or substandard vaccines (a problem announced in Liaoning Province in 2005) which could mask flu symptoms in birds but leave them still contagious;[50] and the possibility that vaccinators themselves could spread the virus on their clothing or shoes unless rigid decontamination procedures are followed.[51]

In another anti-flu initiative, on November 2, 2005, the Chinese government announced an earmark of 2 billion yuan ($420 million) from China's current budget to fight avian flu and the banning of poultry imports from 14 countries affected by avian flu. The Swiss manufacturer of Tamiflu, Roche, also announced it had reached an agreement with China on developing a generic version of Tamiflu.[52]

Despite these preparations, some international health experts quietly continue to question the PRC's transparency on avian flu issues. In late April and June 2005, for instance, PRC officials reported an unknown cause for the suspicious sudden deaths of thousands of migratory birds in western China's Qinghai Lake. In July 2005, a virology team from Hong Kong reported in a scientific journal that their research showed the Qinghai bird deaths were from an H5N1 strain genetically similar to that originating in south China. The Hong Kong report was vigorously criticized as inaccurate by Jia Youling, an official with the PRC Ministry of Agriculture charged with coordinating avian-flu eradication.[53] On June 18, 2005, the *Washington Post* reported that Chinese farmers had been using one of two types of anti-influenza drugs (amantadine, a drug meant for humans) to treat poultry for the H5N1 bird flu virus, potentially rendering the drug ineffective against the virus strain in humans — a story that PRC officials also have denied.[54]

In its anti-flu efforts, China also remains burdened by perennial problems involving local and regional compliance with central government directives. This takes on new dimensions when potential remedies — such as the mandatory destruction of infected poultry flocks — may rob indigent farming families of their principal source of food or cash.

U.S.-PRC Cooperation

President George Bush and PRC President Hu Jintao have discussed greater avian flu coordination on several occasions — during a meeting at the U.N. summit in September 2005 and during Bush's visit to Beijing in November 2005.[55] During the latter visit, the two sides initialed a joint initiative on avian flu, promising to participate in joint research on human and animal virus samples, establish a mechanism to share influenza strains for research purposes, and cooperate actively on a number of regional and international levels, including the WHO, the U.N. Food and Agriculture Organization, and the World Organization of Animal Health. In spite of this

Sino-U.S. agreement, WHO officials on December 30, 2005 announced that as of that date, China still had not shared with international health officials flu virus samples from its infected poultry — a key step in tracking the virus' mutation and devising an effective vaccine.

A this point, the level of cooperation also appears uncertain in another key area of the bilateral agreement — that involving cooperation on "influenza vaccine development." China appears to have advanced on vaccine development — the PRC's State Food and Drug Administration approved clinical trials for a Chinese-developed human avian flu vaccine in November 2005 — and the United States is separately working on a vaccine of its own.

Indonesia[56]

Indonesia is viewed, along with Cambodia, Laos, and Vietnam, as a weak link in the effort to curb an outbreak of avian flu. A lack of resources, expertise, and a slow recognition of the problem has hindered Indonesia's response. Indonesia has a population of some 1.3 billion chickens with as many as 400 million of those in informal settings. Indonesia has resisted mass culling of bird populations. In 2003, when H5N1 was first seen in the bird population, there was not much alarm in Indonesia as the virus was not generally viewed as a significant threat to humans. The virus is now considered endemic in the bird population of Indonesia and outbreaks in birds have so far been reported in 25 out of Indonesia's 33 cities and provinces.[57] Concern grew in June 2005, when Indonesia saw its first human H5N1 fatality. WHO later confirmed H5N1 as the cause of death in July 2005. In October 2005, when a 38-year-old man and two of his children died of the disease in an affluent section of Jakarta, some began to speculate that the virus could spread from person to person, but to date this has not been verified.

There have been a number of questionable reports regarding the number of human cases of H5N1 infection. One report claimed that 85 people had been admitted to hospitals in Indonesia with suspected or confirmed cases of avian flu since the first case in June 2005 (though the man died in June 2005, the cause of death was not attributed to H5N1 until July, as indicated above).[58] However, WHO has only confirmed 16 human cases of H5N1 infection, of whom 11 have died.[59]

While Indonesia was viewed as initially trying to cover up the outbreak, it has more recently moved to address the problem. Plans to stem the spread of the disease, should it mutate and spread more widely among human populations, involve rapid reaction and vaccine distribution. Such an approach is dependent on early detection and reporting by local health officials, and the availability of the resources necessary to treat an outbreak. On December 19, 2005, Indonesia announced a three-year national strategic plan to contain the avian flu virus. The plan will use such measures as culling, vaccination, and community-based surveillance of bird populations. Critics of the plan have pointed out that it does not address birds kept in informal settings.[60] In addition, the government plans to establish a national commission for bird flu control that includes all ministries, private and non-governmental agencies, and the Red Cross.[61]

The Indonesian government appears to be making limited progress in acknowledging and dealing with a large scale outbreak. Foreign Ministry Spokesman Yuri Thamrin has stated "we need international cooperation to fight the virus."[62] Agriculture Minister Anton Apriyanto has indicated that the government will slaughter poultry to stem serious outbreaks. The minister had reportedly earlier stated that the government did not have enough money to compensate farmers for their slaughtered animals. The government reportedly spent $13 million in 2005 to cull infected livestock.[63] According to WHO expert Gina Samaan, Indonesian hospitals are increasingly prepared and "the surveillance system has been enhanced, in the sense that there has been lots of training undertaken to ensure that surveillance of the health department in the provincial and district levels can respond and can initiate an investigation."[64] Eleven companies in Indonesia account for 60% of Indonesian poultry and are reportedly reluctant to allow government monitoring of their birds for fear that they will not be compensated for birds killed to stem an outbreak of the H5N1 avian influenza. Indonesia's poultry industry generated $3.75 billion in revenue in 2004.[65]

Health experts believe Indonesia does not have a sufficient supply of antiviral treatments for a country with more than 200 million people, and where H5N1 is endemic among the bird population. In September, Indonesia's Minister of Health asked for international assistance and expressed concern that her country is not capable of containing the spread of H5N1.[66] Since then, the international community has pledged $140 million in assistance, and the Indonesian Government has allotted just over $60 million for bird flu prevention.[67] WHO officials have also called for countries to donate antiviral drugs to Indonesia. Additionally, Australian Foreign Minister Alexander Downer has warned that Indonesia is not prepared to respond to an avian flu outbreak amongst its human population.

Australia has planned a meeting with Indonesian and WHO officials in Indonesia to strengthen Indonesia's capacity to deal with avian flu. Australia has also pledged funding to Indonesia for the purchase of Tamiflu tablets to treat about 40,000 people.[68] India has also reportedly agreed to provide 1,000 doses, adding to Indonesia's own supply of 10,000 doses.[69]

Reporting indicates that Indonesian officials were aware of bird flu in the bird populations for two years but suppressed the information until humans began to become infected. It has been asserted that "the Indonesian government failed to take measures that could have broken the chain, [of the spread of bird flu] while discouraging research into the outbreak." The outbreak was evidently suppressed due to lobbying by the poultry industry in Indonesia. There are also allegations that the Indonesian government has not funded its announced policy to vaccinate poultry against the virus.[70]

Laos[71]

An outbreak of H5N1 avian flu in poultry was confirmed early 2004, but Laos has had no known cases in humans, according to the WHO. There have been no reports of avian influenza in birds or humans in Laos in 2005.[72] As of June 2005, the Lao government estimated that 60,000 birds had been lost to the infection and another 98,000 to culling. However, this number reflects only documentation from commercial farms; the vast majority of poultry-rearing in Laos takes place in smaller, family-run farms.

Some experts argue that there is an urgent need for foreign health organizations to focus upon and assist Laos, given its proximity to other countries with the disease and the lack of government capacity, particularly its weakness in surveillance. The central and local governments have limited capabilities for collecting and disseminating information, monitoring avian populations, and conducting laboratory analysis to confirm cases of the virus. In addition, according to a U.S. government assessment team that visited Laos, Cambodia, and Vietnam, the country's health care system faces "severe limitations" and would be "quickly overwhelmed" in the event of a large-scale human outbreak.[73] The FAO and the WHO reportedly have strong working relationships with the Lao government.[74] On October 13, 2005, U.S. Secretary of Health and Human Services Michael Leavitt, on a visit to Southeast Asia, signed a cooperation agreement with Lao officials pledging $3.4 million to Laos for controlling outbreaks of avian flu.[75]

Russia[76]

The H5N1 strain spread into Central Asia in 2005 and was first diagnosed in southern Russia (in the Novosibirsk region) as well as in northern Kazakhstan in July 2005. Outbreaks in both countries were attributed to contact between domestic birds and waterfowl migrating from Southeast Asia. There have been no confirmed human cases in Russia. The avian flu spread to eight southern regions of Russia, including two regions bordering the Caspian Sea,[77] but did not spread north toward Moscow.. Besides Russia, avian flu was reported in 2005 in other countries bordering the Black Sea, including Romania, Turkey, and Ukraine, and human cases were reported in Turkey in early 2006. The WHO is concerned about the widening geographical spread of the avian flu into Russia and neighboring countries, because it increases opportunities for humans to catch the virus and for the virus to improve its transmissibility through mutation or reassortment.[78] The WHO's National Flu Center in St. Petersburg announced in August 2005 that it would work more closely with the Vektor Virology Center in southern Russia, which had been monitoring flu viruses among wild migratory birds for several years.

In response to the reports of outbreaks in Russia, the EU in late August raised "serious concerns" that the virus could spread to Western Europe and called on member-states to step up surveillance efforts. It also banned the import of poultry from Russia. Responding to rumors that the avian influenza had spread into western Russia, Germany in October temporarily ordered free-range poultry to be kept indoors, as did the Netherlands in August. Iran, in September 2005, banned the import of Russian wheat as feedstock.[79]

Most observers judged Russia as fairly efficient in identifying avian influenza cases and working with international health organizations, at least at the outset. The areas where the outbreaks occurred were quarantined. No poultry or products were permitted to be exported beyond the areas, poultry in these areas exposed to H5N1 were slaughtered, and many people were examined and immunized. Russia's Deputy Foreign Minister Alexander Yakovenko asserted in early October 2005 that Russia had made a major contribution to countering the spread of avian flu and pandemic flu worldwide.[80] Other observers raised concerns about Russia's ultimate capacity to respond to the spreading virus, or to deal with human cases. They warned that since Russia has devoted few budgetary resources in recent years to improving healthcare, it has not adopted many newer disease-control measures, such as employing fewer and more highly trained staff, using advanced disease-detection equipment, and relying more on primary healthcare. According to one commentator, "pandemic control requires prompt detection of cases and targeted interventions for the first clusters. But it remains doubtful whether Russia has the necessary capacity.... The country's huge size [also] is an obstacle to those services that do function well."[81]

Among measures taken by Russian federal and local officials, Chief Health Inspector Gennadiy Onishchenko issued a directive in August 2005 to implement the May 2005 recommendations of WHO on controlling a possible influenza pandemic. According to WHO criteria, Onishchenko stated, Russia is in the second stage of the avian flu epidemic, when the virus is spreading among fowl and can cause human illness, although it has not become easily transmissible among humans (see Table 1). He called for regional officials to "introduce the necessary corrections into regional plans to prepare for a [human] flu pandemic," including the "allocation of additional funds" for prevention and treatment, and to coordinate these plans with the federal government. In October 2005, he issued instructions to regional and health officials regarding the clinical pattern, differential diagnosis, and prevention and treatment of H5N1 influenza in humans. Regional officials complained that the regions had strained to shoulder the financial burden of compensating owners for the destruction of birds and of other containment measures. Consequently, regional representatives have called on the federal government to provide more funds for responding to possible new outbreaks among poultry, as well as humans. Some observers have also noted that the federal government could have played a greater role in coordinating regional outbreak responses. Analysts have noted that responses in each region were often divergent and not coordinated.[82]

Some Russian doctors and officials have argued that the risk of a pandemic is low, but that the best methods to hedge against such a possibility are better medical care to boost the health of at-risk Russians, flu immunizations for these Russians, and reserve supplies of flu vaccine.[83] They suggest that existing human flu vaccines may help protect the population if H5N1 becomes readily transmissible among humans. In early September 2005, Vladimir Fisinin, the Vice President of the Russian Academy of Agricultural Sciences, called for the Russian government to allocate funds to produce 40 million doses of existing human flu vaccines, as well as 20 million reserve doses. At the same time, the St. Petersburg Institute of Influenza is working with WHO on the development of a human vaccine targeting the H5N1 influenza virus. The Institute in late 2005 reported promising tests in animals, and plans human clinical trials in 2006.

The Moscow newspaper *Nezavisimaya gazeta* in late October 2005 urged the Russian government to also consider buying Tamiflu to treat humans in case of a pandemic.[84]

Russian President Vladimir Putin called in November 2005 for the legislature to approve Russian membership in the U.N.'s FAO, in order to facilitate cooperation with member countries in combating epidemics, including avian influenza. Russia's Federal Service for Veterinary and Plant Control (VPC) in September 2005 proposed that OIE, the European Commission's Health and Consumer Protection Directorate, and U.S. veterinary officials launch a joint program in early 2006 to monitor avian influenza in water fowl as they migrate from places where they spend the winter —Southeast Asia, Africa, northern Australia and Oceania — to Europe, Asia and North and South America. The VPC warned that the H5N1 virus is likely to reappear in southern Russia in Spring 2006 and possibly infect birds migrating towards Central and Eastern Europe.[85]

Thailand[86]

Thailand, among the earliest and hardest hit by the avian flu, has emerged as a leader in fighting the spread of the virus. From the initial 2003 outbreak, 8 of Thailand's 12 reported human cases were fatal.[87] Fourteen of the 22 reported human cases have been fatal to date. As a major poultry exporter, Thailand's economy has suffered significantly from the impact on the industry. After an initially sluggish response, including allegations by the press that government officials covered up evidence of an outbreak[88], the Thai authorities have led the effort to respond to the problem and particularly to facilitate regional cooperation. During a meeting with Prime Minister Thaksin in September 2005, President Bush praised Thailand as a leader in fighting the disease and pledged further U.S. cooperation.

Considerable economic damage from the news of the influenza has spurred Bangkok to address the problem. Thailand's poultry exports, the fourth-largest in the world, bring in over $1 billion annually; the loss this year contributed to a 4.4% year-on-year contraction of the agricultural sector in mid-2005.[89] Both domestic and international demand for chicken fell due to fears of infection. Thailand needs 90 days without outbreaks in order to receive certification from the World Organization for Animal Health (OIE) to resume exporting fresh poultry.[90]

Thai authorities have taken several steps to contain the spread of avian influenza. The Department of Livestock Development, Ministry of

Agriculture and Cooperatives is the focal point for combating the virus, while Department of Disease Control, Ministry of Public Health is also a key player. The National Committee on Avian Influenza Control, under the supervision of a Deputy Prime Minister, was established in 2004 to map out national strategy. As part of the plan, over 40 million birds have been exterminated, and surveillance teams have been deployed throughout the country. In December 2005, the Ministry of Public Health announced that Oseltamivir, an antiviral treatment for influenza, would be produced and distributed to the public at subsidized prices.[91] Bird smuggling from Cambodia was targeted by border authorities.[92] By mid-2005, over 11,000 poultry farms reportedly met the government's biosecurity standards. Thai officials acknowledge, however, that small farms with open-air facilities, which increase the risk of contamination, remain less regulated. Unlike China, Thailand bans the use of H5N1 vaccines in its poultry population. Law enforcement authorities cracked down on illegally imported bird flu vaccines from China; the H5N1 vaccine is prohibited because the government believes that its use in poultry could lead to further mutation of the virus.[93]

After the re-surfacing of the flu in July 2005, the Agriculture and Cooperatives Ministry established guidelines for poultry farmers to get permission from local leaders before moving their flocks. The movement of fowl is considered to be a key concern of livestock officials. Mobile checkpoints were set up in the provinces most affected to enhance scrutiny of such movements.[94] Fighting cocks have been implicated as one of the main transmitters to humans. The sport is intensely popular in Thailand, with up to 30 million spectators annually.[95] The industry, resistant to any form of government control, eventually struck a compromise with the Thai government which allows for the registration of the birds and the stadiums, as well as measures to control their movement.[96]

Thailand has promoted regional cooperation on containing the flu, proposing an ASEAN animal hygienic fund and pledging $300,000 to start the project. The resulting center would enhance cross-border surveillance and control measures, as well as serve as an information distribution center for all ASEAN countries on the spread of the virus[97]. Public Health Minister Suchai Charoenratanakul pledged that Thailand would contribute a minimum of 5% of its own supply to a proposed regional stockpile of antiviral drugs.[98] Thailand and Indonesia pledged to exchange information on influenza prevention and vaccine development. Thailand received one million baht ($25,000) from FAO to set up laboratories and serve as a coordinating center for avian experts, and has received technical assistance from the European Union to improve networking between laboratories working on the avian influenza. Thailand also hosts platforms that are cited as key to the U.S. government response; USAID lists two Bangkok-based organizations as crucial implementing partners.[99]

Turkey[100]

In early January 2006, the WHO confirmed four cases of H5N1 virus in humans; two of them, young siblings, were fatal.[101] The deaths were the first from the virus outside of China and Southeast Asia. Other press reports, citing Turkish officials, claimed up to 15 suspected human cases, most of them children in the eastern rural district of Dogubayazit. WHO officials sent a team to the region for further investigation, and praised the initial response of the Turkish Health Ministry.[102]

Vietnam[103]

WHO reports that there have been 93 confirmed cases — including 42 deaths — of avian influenza in Vietnam since late December 2003. According to USAID, the H5N1 virus is believed to be endemic in Vietnam's waterfowl population. The Vietnamese government estimates the country's total poultry population to be around 250 million birds, including 20 million to 60 million ducks and geese. Between 60% and 70% of the poultry population is raised in "backyard farms," in close proximity to other birds, and the government estimates that 65 per cent of farm households nationwide raise poultry. Poultry generally is sold live in local markets and is slaughtered at home. U.N. agencies have estimated that disease containment, including culling of poultry, have cost the Vietnamese economy an estimated $200 million.[104] The wartime and tsunami supplemental (P.L. 109-13), which the House passed on May 5, 2005 and the Senate on May 10, 2005, provides $25 million to help combat the disease, including approximately $7 million to be used in Vietnam.

In 2005, the Vietnamese government began intensifying its response to the disease by establishing an interagency working group that includes the FAO and WHO. At the local level, inter-ministerial steering committees have been established within the Vietnamese Communist Party's people's committees, which operate throughout the country. However, the quality of inter-ministerial coordination, in addition to the capacity of Vietnam's local institutions to monitor, report, and handle disease outbreaks, have been called into question. The central government in Hanoi is developing a national pandemic preparedness plan, and as of mid-October 2005 had presented a draft to international health agencies and foreign aid donors. Since the first outbreak of avian influenza was reported, over 40 million birds have been culled, though low compensation for farmers appears to have acted as a disincentive for farmers to report signs of infection. In August 2005, Vietnam began a mass poultry vaccination program. In early January 2006, the Ministry of Agriculture and Rural Development (MARD) declared that under the program, all provinces and cities had completed two phases of vaccinations for over 240 million birds. Critics have called Vietnam's previous poultry vaccination programs ineffective. In October 2005, the government signed a bilateral health cooperation agreement with the United States and agreed with a number of U.N. agencies to conduct a joint prevention program.

There are conflicting reports on the willingness of the Vietnamese government to cooperate with international health workers. Many accounts praise the government for responding quickly and cooperatively, particularly in the winter and spring of 2005, when two sets of initial blood tests by Vietnamese and WHO officials indicated that dozens, and perhaps scores, of Vietnamese might have been infected with the virus. Subsequent testing revealed that the initial test results had been false positives.[105] Other accounts, which appear to be in the minority, have charged that the Vietnamese government has been uncooperative with international health agencies, particularly in the first months of the outbreak in 2004.[106]

Issues for Congress

Some experts point out that in order to effectively contain the spread of H5N1 and prepare for pandemic influenza, the U.S. government would need to develop a plan that integrates domestic and international policy. Some of the policy responses may originate domestically, but resonate globally. For example, issues related to U.S. drug policy, such as vaccine technology and intellectual property rights could impact access to antiviral drugs and vaccines in countries where H5N1 is endemic — particularly since some of the most affected countries do not have the capacity to produce or purchase sufficient quantities of the drugs.[107] One article in the Journal of Public Health Policy pointed out that "almost 40% of the world's supply of interpandemic influenza vaccines is used in countries that do not produce their own vaccines."[108]

Concurrently, some domestic issues are impacted by international developments. For example, some are concerned that the United States might not have enough antiviral medication if an influenza pandemic were to occur within the next year since it belatedly ordered Tamiflu (a drug effective in mitigating the course of illness caused by H5N1 infection in most cases). Senator Barack Obama is quoted as expressing concern in an interview that the United States would have to wait for its Tamiflu shipments after Britain, France, and Japan.[109] Some countries in Europe have reportedly ordered enough antiviral medication to treat 20% to 40% of their populations. For example, the Dutch Health Ministry has reportedly ordered enough Tamiflu to treat one-third of the population (5 million doses), and Britain is believed to have ordered enough Tamiflu to treat about 25% of its population (15 million people). Canada reportedly has stocks for just over 5% of its citizens.[110] Current reported U.S. stocks are sufficient to treat slightly more than 1% of all Americans. However, in November 2005, the President announced through the National Strategy for Pandemic Influenza that the United States would procure enough medicine by the end of 2006 to treat 25% of the U.S. population. Below are some issues that particularly impact the most affected countries in Asia, and other parts of the world.

Patent Protections

Intellectual property rights has become an increasingly contentious issue in global health, particularly since companies began threatening to ignore patents for HIV/AIDS treatments. In an effort to expand global access to flu drugs, the United Nations had been encouraging Roche — the patent holder of Tamiflu — to license other companies to produce generic versions of the drug. Roche announced on October 21, 2005 that U.S. pharmaceutical companies could manufacture a generic version of Tamiflu.[111] Legislation introduced in the first session of the 109th Congress aims to permit the United States to invoke a compulsory license and export generic versions of the drug to non-producing countries.[112] Some speculate that Roche has been increasing efforts to license its products in other countries, in part because an Indian pharmaceutical company, Cipla, has threatened to manufacture a generic version of the drug — in spite of Roche's patent rights. Underscoring that Tamiflu is too expensive for many of the least developed countries, a Cipla representative said that the company would sell the generic version of Tamiflu "at a humanitarian price" in developing nations, and not in the United States or Europe.[113] Two Indian pharmaceutical companies are reportedly negotiating with Roche to produce generic versions of Tamiflu.[114] Roche also reached an agreement with a Chinese pharmaceutical company to make the drug.[115]

Health experts predict that patent protections will continue to be a contentious issue as poorer countries seek to protect themselves against virulent diseases. Some analysts contend that Congress faces an issue of whether to help countries where H5N1 is endemic gain greater access to generic versions of Tamiflu and other antivirals if licensed drugs are not accessible. Supporters assert that the precedent for greater access to generics by poorer countries had already been established on December 6, 2005, when World Trade Organization (WTO) members approved changes to the intellectual property agreement making permanent a decision on patents and public health[116]. The General Council decision means that for the first time a core WTO agreement will be amended. The decision directly transforms the August 30, 2003 waiver to Section 31(f) of the Trade-Related Aspects of Intellectual Property Rights (TRIPS)[117]. The waiver permits a country without manufacturing capacity to obtain cheaper generic versions of patented medicines from countries under compulsory licenses. The waiver enables the country to receive generic versions of drugs in situations of "national emergency or other circumstances of extreme urgency."[118] A separate statement describes members' "shared understanding" on how the decision is interpreted and implemented. Particularly, the statement points out that the decision will be used in good faith in order to deal with public health problems and not for industrial or commercial policy objectives.[119] Although the waiver was seen as a tool to enable largely poorer countries to import generic versions of licensed drugs, one piece of legislation proposes that the U.S. Trade Representative inform WTO that the United States declares itself an "eligible importing member" to import pharmaceutical products, largely because Roche is unable to meet the "public health needs" of the United States.[120]

WTO members voted against delineating which drugs should be included in the waiver agreement. Consequently, there is not consensus on which drugs are considered critical in protecting public health. Advocates argue that in the event of a pandemic, the new WTO amendment should apply to antiviral drugs and H5N1 vaccines for use in animals. Opponents are concerned that some might abuse and undermine the agreement by reselling the drugs and vaccines for profit. In the event of a pandemic, Congress might be faced with the decision on whether to support or oppose the export of generic antivirals. Additionally, increased pressure might be placed on Congress to encourage USDA to share with other countries some of its H5N1 vaccine for use in animals.

Global Data Sharing

In spite of Tamiflu stockpiling efforts, it is unknown if the medicine will be broadly useful in treating human H5N1 victims in a pandemic scenario. Some health experts were reportedly alarmed when two patients in Vietnam who were infected with H5N1 and aggressively treated with Tamiflu later died. Some are beginning to question if the recommended dosage should be changed, as doctors reportedly adhered to the recommended regimen when treating the two patients.[121] Health experts point out that more information is needed on patients who have already been treated for H5N1 with Tamiflu. Data from the subjects would help in determining if the drug remains effective in fighting H5N1 and if changes to dosage regimens are required.

Those pressing for greater international data sharing point to new research that might counter previous findings on the limited effectiveness of amantadine. The New York Times reported in September 2005 that researchers found that amantadine was no longer effective against H5N1. WHO reportedly spent $1.3 million to stockpile the drug when it was used during the 1997 H5N1 outbreak. The Times article asserted that in 2005, laboratory research found that all human viral samples of H5N1 were resistant.[122] Before 2000, almost no influenza virus was resistant to the drug. Some experts speculated that viral resistence occurred in part, because China reportedly used amantadine, intended solely for humans, on animals. (See "Affected Countries' Response" section). However, the Wall Street Journal quoted Dr. Shu Yuelong, the Director of China's national influenza laboratory, as stating that preliminary evidence indicates that amantadine might be effective in treating avian influenza in people.[123] Dr. Shu reported that all of the viral samples that have been isolated from patients in China were sensitive to amantadine. Those findings conflicted with previous research on virus samples that were taken from patients in Indonesia and found to be resistant to the drug. The new research has reportedly prompted WHO and other officials to consider whether amantadine might eventually play a role in fighting H5N1. The article underscores that there are currently too few samples to draw any firm conclusions.

Some believe that some countries are intentionally withholding viral samples of H5N1 cases. One article stated that countries with human H5N1 cases do not want to send viral samples to the WHO or other industrialized countries, because they fear the samples will be used to develop up-to-date vaccines which they will not have access to.[124] Others have speculated that China is withholding its samples, because it is trying to produce an H5N1 vaccine.[125]

Some analysts propose that the United States and other countries should vote to provide WHO with enforcement mechanisms. Supporters argue that WHO should be able to force countries to share viral samples. Others contend that Congress should provide greater support and resources to WHO, particularly for strengthening global laboratory and testing capabilities. Skeptics point out that WHO has not provided transparent, detailed data on the adequacy of funds or how funds are spent.

Global Disease Surveillance

A number of analysts have argued that due to insufficient investment in disease surveillance and health care in many of the countries where H5N1 is endemic, a pandemic may progress before it is discovered. In this view, ill-equipped surveillance systems will be slow to determine the source of a pandemic, evaluate the rate of viral transmission, ascertain whether H5N1 has become efficiently transmissible among humans, or rate the effectiveness of anti-flu initiatives. Senate Majority Leader Bill Frist has proposed $1 billion for a real-time international threat detection system.[126]

USAID and other U.S. government officials suspect that the lack of documented human cases of H5N1 in Laos has more to do with inadequate surveillance and reporting systems than an absence of infection.[127] Some health experts believe that H5N1transmission could already be underway in Laos, since surrounding countries have already had human and animal outbreaks. Key U.S. agencies and international organizations have determined that Laos is a country that needs critical prevention, monitoring, and surveillance support in order to prevent full-blown human-to-human transmission of H5N1 that could emerge and sweep across the region without warning.[128]

Some experts have expressed increasing concern about the capacity of poorer countries that have not yet had H5N1 cases to effectively contain the spread of the virus and plan for pandemic influenza, particularly in sub-Saharan Africa. FAO has recently warned that the risk of H5N1 spreading to the Middle East and Africa has markedly increased. FAO is particularly wary of the virus reaching Eastern Africa, as the surveillance capacities and veterinary services in those countries are limited. According to Reuters, a WHO representative declared that an H5N1 outbreak would likely be missed in Africa, as bird nutrition is poor and high mortality among poultry is common. Concurrently, human cluster cases are likely to be missed due to poor surveillance systems. South Africa is reportedly the only country in sub-Saharan Africa to have drawn up a pandemic preparedness plan.[129] Some experts fear that an unabated H5N1 outbreak in East Africa could make the bird flu endemic there. "If the virus were to become endemic in eastern Africa, it could increase the risk that the virus would evolve through mutation or reassortment into a strain that could be transmitted to and between humans."[130]

The press reported on December 20, 2005 that a bird suspected of having contracted H5N1 in Ethiopia, tested negative of the virus.[131] Experts are concerned that birds in Ethiopia and other countries in the Rift Valley, including Kenya, Tanzania, and Uganda, are at particular risk of avian flu infection due to the large numbers of migratory birds that fly to the region during the European winter. Those concerned about insufficient surveillance and diagnostic equipment and expertise, point out that Ethiopia had to use health experts and equipment from Egypt to determine what caused a rash of bird deaths in December 2005. USAID with support from the U.S. Navy Medical Research Unit (NAMRU) in Cairo reportedly provided $15,000 in emergency funding to analyze the viral samples of dead pigeons found in Addis Ababa and the Eastern Somali region for H5N1 infection. Additionally, USAID has reportedly reprogrammed $600,000 from existing surveillance funds for bird flu initiatives in Ethiopia.[132] The funds are to help provide technical assistance to the Ministries of Agriculture and Health, develop laboratory and communications capacity, and procure Personal Protective Equipment for first responders.

Many of the countries in which H5N1 is endemic have complained that they can not afford to implement the strategies recommended by the international community. Furthermore they are hesitant to divert their limited budgets — already struggling to contend with AIDS, child and maternal health, tuberculosis, and other health challenges — to something that might not occur. Advocates of greater assistance to the region, point out that countries with more resources for pandemic planning than neighboring poorer countries have also acknowledged difficulties in responding to the H5N1 threat. A news report cited a South Korean health worker who stated that his country is ill-equipped to respond to a pandemic citing insufficient supplies of medication, hospital beds, and ventilators.[133]

On December 22, 2005, the Senate passed S. 2170, which would help developing countries bolster their disease surveillance programs, and establish fellowships for citizens of those countries to study epidemiology and public health in the United States. Additionally, some in Congress have advocated for greater U.S. spending on fighting the global spread of H5N1 avian flu. Press reports quoted Representatives Henry Hyde and Tom Lantos, Chairman and Ranking Member of the House International Relations Committee respectively, stating concern about the level of funding the Administration proposes to provide for global efforts in FY2006[134]. Advocates assert that the $388 million the Administration requests for international H5N1 initiatives will not be enough to fund the significant amount of assistance needed by countries with H5N1-endemic stocks. Particularly, experts add that the threat of an H5N1 or other influenza pandemic illuminates the neglect that health care systems in many southeast Asian countries have faced over the last couple of decades. Proponents argue that if the United States would increase its funding to support global health care systems the global community could benefit from efficient outbreak reporting and control measures, accurate diagnoses, enhanced case management, and improved disease surveillance and monitoring.

Global Pandemic Planning

Some experts caution that pandemic preparedness plans must extend beyond procuring and stockpiling antiviral drugs and vaccines. In this view, governments must also develop detailed vaccine and treatment distribution plans. Particular attention has been paid to H5N1-affected countries that have communication and infrastructure barriers, especially between urban and rural areas (where many of the backyard poultry farms exist). Many Asian countries have significant income and infrastructure gaps between rural and urban areas. In the rural areas, there are often few hospitals and treatment centers. Equipment can be outdated or lacking. Veterinary and animal health services can be limited. Additionally, in many cases rural governments operate independently from urban governments, which tend to receive larger portions of national resources. Farmers in rural areas may not adhere to government H5N1 initiatives, exacerbating the problem. One infectious disease expert in Hong Kong asserted that the communication problem is particularly acute in China. "I trust and believe the central government has very good intentions, but unfortunately, it is a very big country. At the district, regional levels, the failure to communicate continues."[135]

Responses by East Asian Regional Groupings

As Southeast Asia's major multinational fora, the Association of southeast Asian Nations (ASEAN) has taken some steps to improve transnational coordination in combating the spread of a potential pandemic, and limiting the spread of the H5N1 virus. To this end, ASEAN members have created a number of institutional arrangements, including a Highly Pathogenic Avian Influenza (HPAI) Taskforce, an ASEAN Expert Group on Communicable Diseases, the ASEAN Animal Health Trust Fund, and the ASEAN Plus Three[136] Emerging Infectious Diseases Programme. At the eleventh ASEAN summit in Kuala Lumpur, Malaysia, in December 2005, ASEAN leaders discussed establishing a regional network of stockpiles of antiviral drugs.

Drafting an avian influenza declaration was the single tangible achievement of the inaugural meeting of East Asia's newest regional grouping, the East Asia Summit (EAS), which met in Kuala Lumpur in December 2005 immediately following the ASEAN summit.[137] In their Summit Declaration on Avian Influenza Prevention, Control and Response, EAS leaders committed to "ensure rapid, transparent and accurate ...communications," establish information sharing protocols among member countries and multilateral organizations, create a regional network of stockpiles of antiviral, and to establish regional avian influenza and pandemic preparedness strategies backed by supporting national legislation.

Pandemic planners are warning that no country has the surge capacity to meet national demands for consumer products and medical services for the full term of an influenza pandemic (an estimated six months to a year). The United States, and other industrialized nations, rely on a range of critical products from H5N1-affected countries, such as medical supplies, military parts, and sanitation equipment. These supply chains are replenished "just-in-time" to minimize costs. If an outbreak were to occur, hospitals, food and water systems, and the military could all be vulnerable to interrupted supply due to absenteeism, border closures, and other supply chain disruptions. Therefore, the private sector, as well as national and international trade organizations have been urged to participate in pandemic planning.

Some analysts argue that resources allocated to containing the spread of H5N1 have been insufficient in part, because many countries have funded the response primarily through the Ministries of Agriculture and Health.

Some experts point out that an influenza pandemic will likely impact the animal and health sectors, as well as trade, security, hospitality, and labor. Consequently, they say, governments should develop pandemic plans that utilize the resources of other ministries that are often better funded, such as Ministries of Trade, Tourism, and Commerce. Some analysts note that U.S. officials, such as the U.S. Trade Representative and the Secretary of Commerce should be engaged in U.S. international pandemic influenza planning efforts. Others would like Congress to encourage public-private partnerships that augment U.S. international avian flu and pandemic preparedness efforts.

Combating Bird Flu Among Animals in Affected Countries

Most countries have used mass culling to prevent viral spread when avian influenza outbreaks are detected. However, some countries have not been able to rely on this process as a primary containment measure, because the governments might not have been able to compensate farmers for slaughtering their stocks. Scientists have also found that mass culling is sometimes not feasible when wild birds are involved in transmission. Some health experts assert that there should be more research on more affordable methods of preventing pandemics at their source — in the animals that carry the virus. Strategies such as implementing cleaning days (when all live markets are simultaneously emptied and cleaned), and separating ducks and chickens in live poultry markets may decrease viral transmission among animals. Some countries (including China) propose using vaccination to control avian influenza in poultry. Skeptics warn that animal vaccination is a risky strategy, as it is often difficult to distinguish infected from vaccinated animals, complicating efforts to track the disease. Additionally, vaccination campaigns, if not carried out properly, could result in entrenchment of the disease rather than eradication, further threatening public health.[138]

Cost of Culling

It has been suggested that a global fund should be established to compensate farmers for culling their poultry in countries whose governments can not afford to compensate the farmers. The WHO has already expressed concern that some farmers in poorer countries may not cull their poultry, because their livelihoods depend on poultry farming. For example, Indonesia has carried out only a limited culling drive, because it lacks the funds to compensate farmers.[139] Farmers in some parts of Romania reportedly failed to cull their birds despite government orders to do so. In some affected countries, public and animal health authorities are reluctant to destroy their population's dominant protein source and income. A number of bills, such as H.R. 4062 and its counterpart S. 1821, have been introduced that support the concept of a "Pandemic Fund", which could include funds for farmer compensation.

The World Bank announced that it would provide $500 million in loans to poor countries struggling to fund national avian flu and pandemic preparedness plans —a portion of which could be used to support poor farmers.[140] However, the Bank noted that $1 billion could be needed over the next three years to help countries contain the spread of H5N1. The Asia Development Bank (ADB) also announced that it is prepared to provide at least $470 million to support Asian anti-H5N1 and pandemic preparedness efforts.[141]

Some have suggested that the United States target some foreign aid funds to help the affected governments — including Vietnam, Indonesia, Cambodia, and Laos — cover the cost of compensating individuals and companies for the destruction of their birds. In this view, such assistance could help the image of the United States in the region by demonstrating American concern and could minimize reluctance to slaughter infected flocks. Others would like to see increased assistance to prevent the spread of H5N1 among animals.

Global Economic Impacts

The health and non-health related costs of a global influenza pandemic could be very high, though difficult to estimate. For example, Canadian and Asian hospitality and tourism sectors were considerably impacted during the SARS outbreak. In 2002 and 2003, SARS cost the Asia-Pacific region about $40 billion.[142] Additionally, flights to the region fell by about 45%, crippling the airline and hotel industries. Canada estimated that it lost approximately $1.2 billion, with about $763 million spent on the health-care system.[143] In the event of a flu pandemic, researchers expect Britain, Greece, Spain, Italy, and other countries that rely heavily on tourism, to be most affected economically. One economist estimated that a flu pandemic could force Britain's GDP to fall by 8% or $168 billion (about 95 billion pounds), and result in the loss of almost 1 million jobs (about 3% of all employment).[144]

The World Bank estimates that a global influenza pandemic could cost the global economy about $200 billion in one quarter or $800 billion over a year (about 2% of the global GDP). The Bank based its estimate on the economic losses induced by the SARS pandemic, which caused GDP to fall by 2% in Asia over a three month period in 2003. However, the Bank underscored that it is virtually impossible to accurately determine how much a global influenza pandemic would cost the world, because experts assume that the immediate shock during a flu epidemic could be larger and last longer than SARS. The 1918 pandemic, for example, came in three waves, and spread over two years.[145] Some economists have advised the United States to identify source countries for key imports and develop a detailed plan that would ensure continuity.

Economists point out that an Asian economy crippled by an influenza pandemic could impact the U.S. economy, even if a significant number of Americans was not sickened or killed by H5N1. According to U.S. Trade Representative (USTR) Robert Portman, South Korea and Malaysia are the 7th and 10th largest trading partners for the United States, respectively. The United States earned $72 billion and $40 billion from South Korea and Malaysia, respectively, in 2004. Both countries have had H5N1 cases among their flocks.[146] Additionally, U.S. exports to China, one of the most threatened countries, grew 76 percent between 2000 and 2003, while sales to the rest of the world declined by 9 percent. China is now the sixth largest market for U.S. exports and America's third largest trading partner overall — surpassing Japan in 2003.[147] In 2004, U.S. exports to China grew to $33 billion, more than double the level in 2001.[148] Therefore, any pandemic related disruption of bilateral trade could have a large impact. Alternatively, some economists predict that U.S. poultry exports could increase as countries move to ban imported birds from countries with H5N1-endemic stocks.

CLSA Asia-Pacific Markets, the Asian investment banking arm of Crédit Agricole of France, estimates that H5N1 has already cost the region between $8 billion and $12 billion, citing the prolonged poultry ban by the European Union from eight Asian countries and the death or destruction of some 140 million chickens and other poultry. The Prime Minister of Thailand stated that the avian flu has already cost his country some $1.09 billion, in addition to the $55.78 million the government paid to farmers for a mass chicken cull.[149]

Some analysts caution that Congress should be prepared to respond to the impact that potential fluctuations in supply and demand from key Asian markets might have on the U.S. economy. Particularly, some would like

Congress to direct the U.S. Trade Representative to prepare a report that comprehensively analyzes the potential economic gains and losses to the U.S. economy in a pandemic scenario due to changes in Asia's economy. Experts point out that the Congressional Budget Office (CBO) report *A Potential Influenza Pandemic: Possible Macroeconomic Effects and Policy Issues* focuses on possible supply and demand changes in the U.S. economy if an H5N1 pandemic were to reach the United States.[150] The Wall Street Journal reported that the U.S. poultry industry currently exports about 15% of its chicken meat annually, earning $2.2 billion in 2004. The article asserted that some poultry-industry executives are concerned that importing countries might reject poultry from states that have vaccinated the animals.[151] Consequently, many executives in the poultry industry are opposed to vaccinating chickens intended for export. Some would like Congress to require USDA to present clear guidelines on how and when poultry would have to be vaccinated.

Global Biosafety

In October 2005, scientists reported that the 1918 influenza pandemic that had killed between 20 million and 50 million people worldwide may have emerged from an avian flu strain. Health experts have debated whether the genetic sequence of the 1918 influenza should be published. Some were concerned that the information could be used to construct a biological weapon. However, other scientists argued that sharing such important findings is critical to efficiently identifying dangerous viruses, and to finding ways to disable them. Ultimately, the genetic sequence was published.[152] Dr. Anthony Fauci, Director of the National Institute of Allergy and Infectious Diseases, and Dr. Julie Gerberding, Director of the CDC, said in a joint statement, "The new studies could have an immediate impact by helping scientists focus on detecting changes in the evolving H5N1 virus that might make widespread transmission among humans more likely." Furthermore, the HHS National Science Advisory Board for Biosecurity "voted unanimously that the benefits [to making the results public] outweighed the risk that it would be used in a nefarious manner."[153] However, the Administration acknowledged that the influenza virus could be used as a biological weapon and added the virus to the Select Agent list on October 20, 2005.[154] Congress authorized the Select Agent program in the late 1990s to track the movement of certain bacteria and viruses that could potentially be used as bioterrorist weapons.[155]

Health specialists caution that lab safety must be a top priority as other countries begin to develop their own research and vaccine capacities. Some are closely watching Taiwan in its effort to build its own influenza vaccine factory.[156] Japan, already accomplished in viral research, is reportedly helping Vietnam build a biosafety lab to work with the influenza virus.[157] If global influenza vaccine production is to increase, disease experts caution that some form of oversight must first be established. Some scientists advocate the development of an international influenza research facility. Supporters envision a global laboratory that could rapidly identify influenza threats, and produce appropriate vaccines. It also could, they say, streamline existing flu monitoring systems. Opponents of this idea believe that current technology, such as the WHO's Internet-based FluNet, is fully capable of obtaining the same goal. Furthermore, critics believe that scientists might lose interest in sharing viral samples, if they believe their analytical and research capacities will be taken away.[158]

S. 1873, *The Biodefense and Pandemic Vaccine and Drug Development Act*, would address production of pandemic products. The bill would authorize funding for surge capacity of manufacturing vaccines. It would also authorize funding for research and development of flu vaccines, counter measures, and pandemic products.

APPENDIX

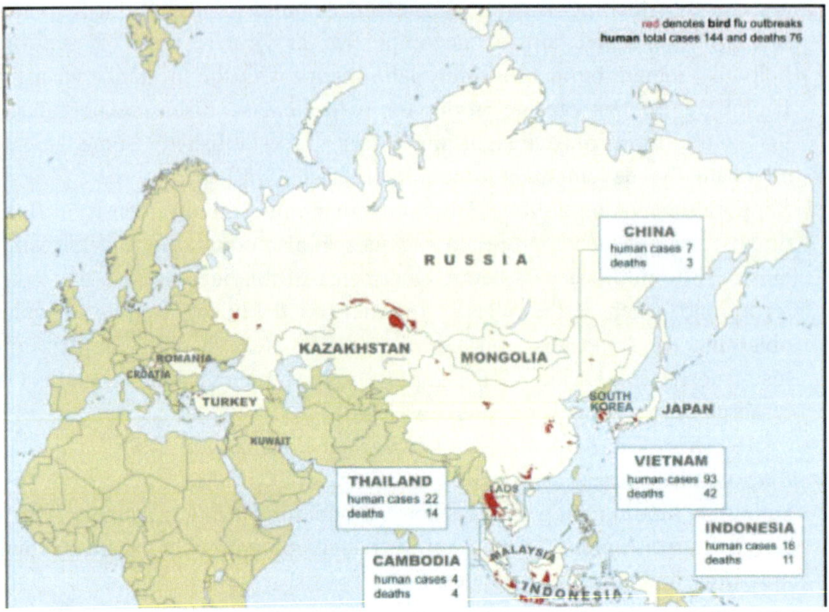
red denotes bird flu outbreaks
human total cases 144 and deaths 76
RUSSIA
CHINA
human cases 7
deaths 3
KAZAKHSTAN
MONGOLIA
ROMANIA
CROATIA
TURKEY
KUWAIT
SOUTH KOREA
JAPAN
VIETNAM
human cases 93
deaths 42
THAILAND
human cases 22
deaths 14
LAOS
INDONESIA
human cases 16
deaths 11
MALAYSIA
CAMBODIA
human cases 4
deaths 4
INDONESIA

Source: Information Based on the World Health Organization (WTO) website, and the World Organization for Animal Health (OIE) website. Adapted by CRS. (K Yancey 1/6/06).

Figure 1. Map of Human and Animal H5N1 Cases

Table 2. WHO Pandemic Phases

Phase	Description	Overarching Public Health Goals
Interpandemic Period		
Phase 1	No new influenza virus strains have been detected in humans. A virus strain that has caused human infection may be present in animals. If so, the risk of human infection is considered to be low.	Strengthen global influenza pandemic preparedness at the global, regional and national levels.
Phase 2	No new influenza virus strains have been detected in humans. However, a circulating animal influenza virus strain poses a substantial risk of human disease.	Minimize the risk of transmission to humans; detect and report such transmission rapidly if it occurs.
Pandemic Alert Period		
Phase 3	Human infection(s) with a new strain, but no human-to-human spread, or at most rare instances of spread to a close contact.	Ensure rapid characterization of the new virus strain, and early detection, notification and response to additional cases.
Phase 4	Small cluster(s) with limited human-to-human transmission, but spread is highly localized, suggesting that the virus is not well adapted to humans.	Contain the new virus within limited foci or delay spread to gain time to implement preparedness measures, including vaccine development.
Phase 5	Larger cluster(s), but human to human spread still localized, suggesting that the virus is becoming increasingly better adapted to humans, but may not yet be fully transmissible (substantial pandemic risk).	Maximize efforts to contain or delay spread, to possibly avert a pandemic, and to gain time to implement pandemic response measures.
Pandemic Period		
Phase 6	Pandemic: increased and sustained transmission in the general population	Minimize the impact of the pandemic.

Source: World Health Organization.

Table 3. FY2006 Emergency Supplemental Request ($ millions)

AGENCY	ACTIVITIES	AMOUNT
Department of Health and Human Services	Increase vaccine manufacturing capacity so that 25% of Americans would have access to antiviral medication, and the entire U.S. population would have access to pandemic influenza vaccines within a six-month period.	6,700.0
Department of Agriculture	Research and development, domestic surveillance and diagnosis of live bird markets, wildlife and bird flyways, smuggling and waterfowl, planning and preparedness training and modeling of scenarios, and the production of 40 million doses of animal vaccine.	91.4
Department of Defense	Purchasing avian influenza vaccines, increasing world wide surveillance of the virus, and upgrading surveillance, laboratory, information management equipment. Additionally, $10 million of the $130 million is intended to assist military partner nations in procuring protective equipment, laboratory diagnostic equipment, portable field assay testing equipment surveillance, and essential communication equipment.	130.0
Department of Homeland Security	Pandemic scenario modeling, personal protective equipment, private sector pandemic assistance planning, and exercises and training for DHS frontline staff.	47.3
Department of the Interior	For the U.S. Geological Survey (USGS), the U.S. Fish and Wildlife Service, the National Park Service, and other Federal agencies to begin an interagency effort to detect avian influenza in wild birds, with an initial focus on early detection activities in Alaska and coastal areas.	11.6
Department of State	International response coordination, including foreign governments and non-governmental organizations, diplomatic outreach, exchanges of U.S. and foreign medical personnel, and for avian and pandemic influenza health support and protection of U.S. government employees and families at U.S. missions overseas. $20 million of the funds would be reserved for the potential evacuation of U.S. government personnel and dependents from overseas missions.	38.5
Department of Veterans Affairs	Increasing avian influenza surveillance programs and establishing real-time surveillance data links with CDC.	27.0
USAID	Pre-position supplies and equipment to prevent and control the spread of avian influenza(within one year of receiving funds); increase awareness of risks and appropriate behaviors to reduce transmission among humans and animals; improve surveillance and response; and accelerate international planning and preparedness. $2 million of the funds are reserved for Russia and Eastern Europe.	131.5
GRAND TOTAL		7,177.3

Source: Prepared by CRS from FY2006 Emergency Request.

Table 4. FY2006 Appropriations Providing Funds for Global Initiatives

<table>
<tr><th>Legislation</th><th>FY2006 Senate Appropriations</th><th>FY2006 House Appropriations</th></tr>
<tr><td>H.R. 3010, Labor, HHS, Education</td><td>$60 million for global surveillance.</td><td>$36.5 million to combat the spread of the avian flu in Asia, and to enhance global surveillance and response network for infectious diseases.</td></tr>
<tr><td colspan="3">H.Rept. 109-337 provides $183.5 million for the Public Health and Social Services Emergency Fund (PHSSEF), of which $120 million would be available until expended. Presented to the President for signature on December 28, 2005.</td></tr>
<tr><td>P.L. 109-102, Foreign Operations</td><td>$10 million, control the spread of the avian flu.</td><td>No similar language.</td></tr>
<tr><td colspan="3">P.L. 109-1 02 provides $25 million for strengthening international surveillance, reporting, and response capacity.</td></tr>
<tr><td>H.R. 2863, Department of Defense</td><td>$33 million, avian flu global surveillance;</td><td>No similar language.</td></tr>
<tr><td colspan="3">H.Rept. 109-359 provides $3.8 billion for avian flu initiatives, of which $3.3 billion is directed to the Public Health and Social Services Emergency Fund. $267 million of the $3.3 billion is reserved for international initiatives, disease surveillance, vaccine registries, research, and clinical trials. An additional $500 million is reserved for international assistance, monitoring and tracking, and research and development. The conference report, H.Rept. 109-359, Emergency Supplemental Appropriations to Address Hurricanes in the Gulf of Mexico and Pandemic Influenza, provides $3.8 billion for avian influenza initiatives. Specifically, the bill directs $3.3 billion to PHSSEF, $131.5 million to USAID, $130 million to the Department of Defense, $71.5 million to APHIS, $47.3 million to the Department of Homeland Security, $20 million to FDA, $27 million to the Department of Veterans Affairs, $31 million to the Department of State, and $11.6 million to the Department of the Interior. Presented to the President for signature on December 28, 2005.</td></tr>
</table>

Source: Prepared by CRS from FY2006 appropriations legislation.

Table 5. Country Allocations for FY2005 Supplemental

COUNTRY	CDC FUNDING	USAID FUNDING
Vietnam	$2.634 million	$ 3.45 million
Indonesia	$0.25 million	$ 3.15 million
Cambodia	$ 1.858 million	$ 2.25 million
Laos	$ 1.858 million	$ 1.60 million
China	$0.00	$ 0.50 million
Regional	$3.35 million	$ 2.75 million
TOTAL	$9.95 million	$13.7 million

Sources: USAID Press Release, October 27, 2005 and CDC Washington Office, November 8, 2005. CDC Funding reflects spending from FY2005 Emergency Supplemental. USAID Funding includes reallocated funds from other programs.

Table 6. International Partnership on Avian and Pandemic Influenza (IPAPI) Core Principles

1. International cooperation to protect the lives and health of our people;
2. Timely and sustained high-level global political leadership to combat avian and pandemic influenza;
3. Transparency in reporting of influenza cases in humans and in animals caused by strains that have pandemic potential, to increase understanding, preparedness and, especially to ensure rapid and timely response to potential outbreaks;
4. Immediate sharing of epidemiological data and samples with the World Health Organization (WHO) and the international community to detect and characterize the nature and evolution of any outbreaks as quickly as possible, by utilizing, where appropriate, existing networks and mechanisms;
5. Rapid reaction to address the first signs of accelerated transmission of H5N1 and other highly pathogenic influenza strains so that appropriate international and national resources can be brought to bear;
6. Prevent and contain an incipient epidemic through capacity building and in-country collaboration with international partners;
7. Work in a manner complementary to and supportive of expanded cooperation with and appropriate support of key multilateral organizations (WHO, Food and Agriculture Organization, World Organization for Animal Health);

8. Timely coordination of bilateral and multilateral resource allocations; dedication of domestic resources (human and financial); improvements in public awareness; and development of economic and trade contingency plans;
9. Increased coordination and harmonization of preparedness, prevention, response and containment activities among nations, complementing domestic and regional preparedness initiatives and encouraging where appropriate the development of strategic regional initiatives;
10. Actions based on the best available science.

Source: State Department Press Release, "U.S. Launches International Partnership on Avian and Pandemic Influenza." September 22, 2005. [http://www.state.gov/r/pa/prs/ps/2005/53865.htm]

References

[1] For a list of past avian flu outbreaks see CRS Report RS21747, *Avian Influenza: Agricultural Issues*, by Jim Monke.

[2] WHO, "Avian Influenza — New Areas with Infection in Birds — Update 34," *Disease Outbreak News*, Oct. 13, 2005, at [http://www.who.int/csr/don/en/].

[3] Osterholm, Michael, "Pandemic Influenza: A Harbinger of Things to Come." Presentation at the Woodrow Wilson International Center for Scholars, September 19, 2005. [http://www.wilsoncenter.org/index.cfm?fuseaction=news.itemandnews_id=145329]

[4] HHS Pandemic Influenza Plan, November 2005, [http://www.hhs.gov/pandemicflu/plan/]. For more information on issues related to domestic efforts to address H5N1 and pandemic influenza preparedness, see CRS Report RL33145, *Pandemic Influenza: Domestic Preparedness Efforts*, by Sarah A. Lister.

[5] To date, H5N1 has been identified among birds in Cambodia, China, Croatia, Indonesia, Japan, Kazakhstan, Korea, Laos, Malaysia, Mongolia, Romania, Russia, Thailand, Turkey, and Vietnam. A bird in Britain was diagnosed with H5N1, however it was an isolated case found in an imported bird that died in quarantine. World Organization for Animal Health (OIE), "Update on Avian Influenza in Animals." December 21, 2005. [http://www.oie.int/eng/en_index.htm]

[6] WHO, *Cumulative Number of Confirmed Human Cases of Avian Influenza A/H5N1*, January 9, 2006. [http://www.who.int/csr/disease/avian_influenza/country/en/]

[7] For more information on the domestic response to H5N1, see CRS Report RL33145, *Pandemic Influenza: Domestic Preparedness Efforts*, by Sarah A. Lister, and CRS Report RS21747, *Avian Influenza: Agricultural Issues*, by Jim Monke.

[8] The FY2006 Defense, Disaster Assistance, and Avian Flu Preparedness Appropriations conference report, H.Rept. 109-359, contains \$3.8 billion for avian influenza initiatives. \$3.3 billion of the \$3.8 billion is directed to the Department of Health and Human Services (HHS) (of which \$267 million is reserved for international initiatives, disease surveillance, vaccine registries, research, and clinical trials). An additional \$500 million is reserved for international assistance, monitoring and tracking, and research and development, of which \$131.5 million is directed to USAID, \$130 million to the Department of Defense, \$71.5 million to the Department of Agriculture, \$47.3 million to the Department of Homeland Security, \$20 million to FDA, \$27 million to the Department of Veterans Affairs, \$31 million to the Department of State, and \$11.6 million to the Department of the Interior.

[9] CQ Today, "*Bush Flu Spending Request Meets Resistance from House Republicans.*" November 8, 2005. [http://www.cq.com]

[10] FY2006 Emergency Request for Avian and Pandemic Influenza Preparedness. [http://www.whitehouse.gov/omb/budget/amendments/supplemental_11_01_05.pdf]

[11] Report from Country Planning Visits, "U.S. Government Emergency Response to Avian Influenza: A Plan of Action for Vietnam, Laos, and Cambodia." July 11-24, 2005. This report was provided to CRS by USAID.

[12] Interviews with CDC staff, October 13, 2005 and November 1, 2005.

[13] USAID Fact Sheet "Avian Influenza Preparedness, Response, and Containment." October 27, 2005. [http://www.usaid.gov].

[14] The State Department also implements influenza pandemic preparedness initiatives through the Office of International Health Affairs (OES/IHA), which works with agencies throughout the U.S. government to facilitate policy-making regarding bioterrorism and health security, environmental health, infectious diseases (e.g., SARS, Avian Influenza, Pandemic Influenza, Polio), health in post-conflict

situations, and surveillance and response. [http://www.state.gov/g/oes/c1874.htm].

[15] USDA, Transcript of Technical Briefing regarding Avian Influenza. October 26, 2005. [http://www.usda.gov/birdflu]

[16] GEIS website, [http://www.geis.fhp.osd.mil/].

[17] DoD, Global Emerging Infections System Annual Report Fiscal Year 2004. [http://www.geis.fhp.osd.mil/GEIS/aboutGEIS/annualReports/GEIS_AR_04.pdf].

[18] DoD, Global Emerging Infections System Annual Report Fiscal Year 2004. [http://www.geis.fhp.osd.mil/GEIS/aboutGEIS/annualReports/GEIS_AR_04.pdf].

[19] This section prepared by Rhoda Margesson, Analyst in Foreign Affairs.

[20] For more information on the Global Outbreak Alert and Response Network, see [http://www.who.int/csr/outbreaknetwork].

[21] The WHO influenza pandemic preparedness Home Page is at [http://www.who.int/csr/disease/influenza/pandemic/en/index.html].

[22] See WHO, Department of Communicable Disease Surveillance and Response Global Influenza Programme, "Responding to the Avian Influenza Pandemic Threat: Recommended Strategic Actions," WHO/CDS/CSR/GIP2005.8.

[23] WHO, "Donation of three million treatments of oseltamivir to WHO will help early response to an emerging influenza pandemic." August 24, 2005. [http://www.who.int/mediacentre/news/releases/2005/pr36/en/index.html].

[24] Roche, "Roche donates 3 million treatments of antiviral Tamiflu to the WHO for use in an influenza pandemic." August 24, 2005. [http://www.roche.com/med-cor-2005-08-24]

[25] United Nations, "U.N. Establishes New Emergency Fund," December 16, 2005. [http://www.irinnews.org]

[26] See FAO avian influenza home page at [http://www.fao.org/ag/againfo/subjects/en/ health/diseases-cards/special_avian.html].

[27] See OIE avian flu home page at [http://www.oie.int/eng/AVIAN_INFLUENZA/ home.htm]

[28] Interview with FAO official, October 31, 2005.

[29] World Bank Press Release, "New Global Program to Deal with Avian Flu." November 4, 2005. [http://www.worldbank.org]

[30] UN News Service, "Bird flu: UN-sponsored conference draws up six-point action plan." November 9, 2005. [http://www.un.org/apps/news/]

[31] The World Bank Group, "Partners Meeting on Avian Influenza and Human Pandemic Influenza." [http://www.worldbank.org]

[32] UN News Service, "Bird flu: UN-sponsored conference draws up six-point action plan." November 9, 2005. [http://www.un.org/apps/news/]

[33] The American Society of International Law, *SARS and International Law,* April 2003, see [http://www.asil.org/insights].

[34] The revised International Health Regulations, approved by the World Health Assembly on May 23, 2005, are available at [http://www.who.int/csr/ihr/en/].

[35] If a State makes a reservation that is compatible with the "object and purpose of IHR (2005)" and at least one-third of other States have not objected to the reservation within six months of notification, the revised IHR will enter into force for that State, subject to its reservation. See WHO, "Frequently Asked Questions About IHR," at [http://www.who.int/csr/ihr/howtheywork/faq].

[36] See WHO, "Frequently Asked Questions About IHR," at [http://www.who.int/csr/ihr/howtheywork/faq].

[37] "The Front Lines in the Battle Against Avian Flu Are Running Short of Money," *New York Times*. October 9, 2005.

[38] OIE, Update on Avian Influenza in Animals, January 9, 2006. [http://www.oie.int/]

[39] This section prepared by Thomas Lum, Specialist in Asian Affairs, 7-7616.

[40] "U.S., Cambodian Health Ministers Sign Deal on Bird Flu Cooperation," *Agence France Press*. October 11, 2005.

[41] "Cambodia Needs $18 Million for Bird Flu Fight — UN," *Reuters*, December 16, 2005.

[42] This section was prepared by Kerry Dumbaugh, Specialist in Asian Affairs, 7-7683.

[43] As of January 1, 2006, there were 7 confirmed cases of avian flu and 3 deaths in China.

[44] For more on SARS — Severe Acute Respiratory Syndrome — see CRS Report RL32227, SARS, Avian Flu, and other Challenges for China's Political, Social, and Economic Transformation.

[45] According to the U.S. Centers for Disease Control and Prevention. See website at [http://www.cdc.gov/flu/avian/outbreaks/asia.htm].

[46] *Beijing Liaowang* in Chinese. Translated on September 26, 2005, in FBIS, CPP20051018050001.

[47] PRC Ministry of Health, "Preparations and Plan for an Influenza Pandemic Emergency," September 28, 2005, translated in FBIS, CPP20051012335002 (October 12, 2005).

[48] Cody, Edward, "China to vaccinate billions of birds; campaign aims to stem avian flu," *Washington Post*, November 16, 2005, p. A15.

[49] Fountain, Henry, "How to vaccinate 14 billion birds," *The New York Times*, November 20, 2005, p. 2.

[50] Sipress, Alan, bird flu experts warn against bad vaccines; improper poultry inoculation may spread virus," *Washington Post*, November 22, 2005, p. A24.

[51] McNeil, Donald Jr., "Health experts fear Chinese flu vaccination plan could backfire," *The New York Times,* November 20, 2005, p. 12.

[52] Wright, Tom, "*Roche to Let Chinese Producer Make Flu Drug.*" New York Times, December 13, 2005.

[53] The independent virology team was from the University of Hong Kong and included Dr. Guan Yi, a co-author of the scientific report published in *Nature* magazine on July 7, 2005. For reference to PRC official Jia Youling's comments, see Sipress, Alan, "China has not shared crucial data on bird flu outbreaks, officials say," in the *Washington Post*, July 19, 2005, p. A15.

[54] *Washington Post*, June 18, 2005, p. A01. Some sources also have suggested that the virus' apparent new resistance to known drugs may be the result of renegade pharmaceutical labs in China dispensing the wrong anti-viral medications, raising additional questions about the PRC government's ability to exert control over a potential pandemic. *International Herald Tribune*, July 5, 2005, p. 3.

[55] King Jr., Neil, "Hu pledges efforts to ease U.S. strains — ," *Asian Wall St. Journal*, September 15, 2005, p. A1.

[56] This section prepared by Bruce Vaughn, Analyst in Asian Affairs, 7-3144.

[57] "Indonesia Set to Form National Commission for Bird Flu Control," Thai News Service. January 10, 2006.

[58] "Indonesia Reduces Confirmed Bird Flu Death Toll to 3 from 6," *AFX Asia*. October 6, 2005.

[59] WHO, *Confirmed Human Cases of Avian Influenza A (H5N1).* Accessed on December 30, 2005. [http://www.who.int/csr/disease/avian_influenza/country/en/]

[60] "Toll UP but Indonesia Ready for Bird Flu," *ISI Emerging Markets*. January 2, 2006.

[61] "Indonesia Set to Form National Commission for Bird Flu Control," Thai News Service. January 10, 2006.

[62] "Indonesia Calls for Intl Cooperation to Combat Bird Flu," *Dow Jones Newswire*. Sept. 30, 2005.

[63] Alan Sipress, "Indonesia Warns of Possible Bird Flu Epidemic," *Washington Post*. September 21, 2005.

[64] "Indonesia Making Progress in Fight Against Bird Flu - WHO," *AFX Asia*. September 30, 2005.

[65] Phelim Kyne and Fitri Wulandari, "Indonesian Poultry Cos Hobble Avian Flu Control Ops," *Dow Jones Newswires*. October 5, 2005.

[66] Reuters, "Indonesia says bird flu outbreak may become epidemic." September 21, 2005. [http://www.alertnet.org].

[67] "Indonesia Set to Form National Commission for Bird Flu Control," Thai News Service. January 10, 2006.

[68] Nicholas Zaminska, "Asian Nations Start Critical Bird Flu Preparations," *The Wall Street Journal*. October 3, 2005.

[69] Eaton, Dan and Telly Nathalia, "Indonesia says bird flu outbreak may become epidemic." Reuters. September 21, 2005. [http://www.alertnet.org/thenews/newsdesk/JAK58836.htm].

[70] Alan Sipress, "Indonesia Neglected Bird Flu Until Too Late," *The Washington Post*, October 20, 2005.

[71] This section prepared by Thomas Lum, Specialist in Asian Affairs, 7-7616.

[72] "WHO Urges Laos to Prepare for Deadly Human Version of Bird Flu," *Agence France Presse*, August 27, 2005.

[73] "U.S. Government Emergency Response to Avian Influenza: A Plan for Vietnam, Laos and Cambodia: Report from Country Planning Visits," July 2005.

[74] "WHO Urges Laos to Prepare for Deadly Human Version of Bird Flu," *Agence France Presse*. August 27, 2005

[75] "Intl Donors Pledge More Than $17M to Help Southeast Asia Combat Bird Flu," *Forbes.com*. October 13, 2005.

[76] This section prepared by Jim Nichol, Specialist in Russian and Central Asian Affairs, 7-2289.

[77] The eight administrative areas are the Astrakhan, Chelyabinsk, Kurgan, Novosibirsk, Omsk, and Tyumen oblasts (regions), the Kalmyk republic, and the Altay kray (territory).

[78] World Health Organization. *Geographical Spread of H5N1 Avian Influenza in Birds: Situation Assessment and Implications for Human Health, Update 28*, August 18, 2005.

[79] *Agence France Presse*, August 22, 2005; *Foreign Broadcast Information Service* (FBIS), September 3, 2005, Doc. No. IAP-11012.
[80] *The Lancet*, August 27-September 2, 2005, p. 689; *Interfax*, October 4, 2005.
[81] *The Lancet*, August 27-September 2, 2005, p. 689.
[82] *FBIS*, August 18, 2005, Doc. No. CEP-19027.
[83] *FBIS*, September 13, 2005, Doc. No. CEP-346004.
[84] *ITAR-TASS*, October 23, 2005; *ITAR-TASS,* October 27, 2005; *FBIS*, October 24, 2005, Doc. No. CEP-346001; December 6, 2005, Doc. No. CEP-346002.
[85] *FBIS*, September 7, 2005, Doc. No. CEP-27067.
[86] This section prepared by Emma Chanlett-Avery, Analyst in Asian Affairs, 7-7748.
[87] WHO, *Cumulative Number of Confirmed Human Cases of Avian Influenza A/H5N1 Reported to WHO*, December 7, 2005. [http://www.who.int/csr/disease/avian_influenza/country/en/].
[88] "Thai Authorities Should Take Strong Action Against Bird Flu," *Bangkok Post* editorial. October 4, 2005.
[89] "Bird Flu: Asian Contagion?" *Economist Intelligence Unit*. July 25, 2005.
[90] "Thailand Has First Avian Flu Outbreaks in 3 Months," CIDRAP News at [http://www.cidrap.umn.edu]. July 11, 2005.
[91] "Thai Public Health Minister Announced that Thailand Can Produce Oseltamivir," *Thai News Service*. December 8, 2005.
[92] "Squawking at the Bird Flu Warning," *Los Angeles Times*. September 1, 2005.
[93] "Thailand Cracks Bird Flu Vaccine Smuggling Syndicate," *BBC Monitoring Asia Pacific*. September 20, 2005.
[94] "Avian Flu - Fresh Outbreak," *Bangkok Post*. July 14, 2005.
[95] "Squawking at the Bird Flu Warning," *Los Angeles Times*. September 1, 2005.
[96] "Ministry cuts Deal of Fighting Cock Zoning," *Bangkok Post*. July 15, 2005.
[97] "Thailand Proposes Regional Bird Flu Control Center," *Thai News Service*. September 27, 2005.
[98] "Bird Flu Pandemic Risk 'Very High'," *CNN.com*. October 11, 2005.
[99] "U.S. Government Emergency Response to Avian Influenza: A Plan of Action for Vietnam, Laos, and Cambodia - Report from Country Planning Visits July 11-24, 2005. " United States Agency for International Development.

[100] This section prepared by Emma Chanlett-Avery, Analyst in Asian Affairs, 7-7748.

[101] WHO, *Cumulative Number of Confirmed Human Cases of Avian Influenza A/H5N1* January 7, 2006. [http://www.who.int/csr/don/2006_01_07/en/index.html]

[102] "Bird Flu Spreads Across Turkey," *CNN News Online.* January 9, 2006.

[103] This section prepared by Mark Manyin, Specialist in Asian Affairs, 7-7653.

[104] USAID, "U.S. Government Emergency Response to Avian Influenza: A Plan of Action for Vietnam, Laos and Cambodia. Report from Country Planning Visits," July 11-24, 2005.

[105] See, for instance, Nicholas Zamiska, "Pandemic Watch: Inside U.N. Agency, Flu Data Sparked A Tense Debate," *The Wall Street Journal*, October 18, 2005.

[106] See, for instance, Adrian Levy and Cathy Scott-Clark, "Flu on the Wing," *The Guardian*, October 15, 2005.

[107] For more information on these issues see CRS Report RL31145, *Pandemic Influenza: Domestic Preparedness Efforts*, by Mark Gurevitz.

[108] Fedson, David, "Preparing for Pandemic Vaccination: An International Policy Agenda for Vaccine Development." *Journal of Public Health Policy 2005*, Volume 26, Issue 1, April 2005. p.11.

[109] Harris, Gardiner, "Officials May Spend Billions to Stockpile Influenza Drug." New York Times, October 7, 2005.

[110] Ibid.

[111] Alonso-Zaldivar, Ricardo, "Roche agrees to generic version of Tamiflu drug." *Baltimore Sun*, October 21, 2005. [http://www.baltimoresun.com].

[112] H.R. 4392, *To provide for the importation of pharmaceutical products under a compulsory license as provided for under the World Trade Organization.*

[113] McNeil Jr., Donald, "Indian Company to Make Generic Version of Flu Drug Tamiflu." New York Times. October 14, 2005. [http://www.nytimes.com].

[114] Jack, Andrew, "India drugs groups in Tamiflu talks." Financial Times. December 12, 2005. [http://news.ft.com/home/us/]

[115] Wright, Tom, "Roche to Let Chinese Producer Make Flu Drug." *New York Times*. December 13, 2005. [http://nytimes.com]

[116] WTO, "Members OK amendment to make health flexibility permanent." December 6, 2005. [http://www.wto.org/english/news_e/pres05_e/pr426_e.htm]
[117] Article 31(f) of the TRIPS Agreement says that production under compulsory licensing must be predominantly for the domestic market. The concern was that this could limit the ability of countries that cannot make pharmaceutical products from importing cheaper generics from countries where pharmaceuticals are patented.
[118] For more information on this issue see CRS Report RS21609, *The WTO, Intellectual Property Rights, and the Access to Medicines of Controversy*, by Ian F. Fergusson.
[119] WTO, "Members OK amendment to make health flexibility permanent." December 6, 2005. [http://www.wto.org/english/news_e/pres05_e/pr426_e.htm]
[120] H.R. 4392, *To provide for the importation of pharmaceutical products under a compulsory license as provided for under the World Trade Organization.*
[121] Chang, Alicia, "Bird Flu Victims Die After Drug Resistence." Washington Post. December 21, 2005. [http://www.washingtonpost.com]
[122] Rosenthal, Elisabeth, "Two Studies Find Flu Treatments Fall Far Short." September 22, 2005. [http://www.nytimes.com].
[123] Zamiska, Nicholas, "Scientists Says Bird-Flu Virus Appears to Be Stable in China; No Signs that Avian Strain Is Easily passed by People; Old Drug Shows Promise." December 12, 2005.
[124] Globe and Mail, "Chinese officials haven't shared samples of H5N1: experts." November 18, 2005. [http://www.theglobeandmail.com].
[125] China Daily, "China: Bird flu vaccine for human use developed." November 15, 2005. [http://www.chinadaily.com.cn/english/doc/2005-11/15/content_494593_3.htm].
[126] Honorable Bill Frist website, "First Addresses National Press Club on Avian Flu —Pandemic: The Economy Killer." December 8, 2005. The Senate passed S. 2170 on December 22, 2005.
[127] Interview with USAID official, October 11, 2005.
[128] Ibid.
[129] Reuters, "Bird Flu in Africa Could Swamp Health Systems: WHO." November 27, 2005. [http://www.nlm.nih.gov/medlineplus/news/fullstory_27731.html]
[130] "UN agency says risk of bird flu spreading to Middle East, Africa rises markedly." U.N. News Center, October 19, 2005.

[http://www0.un.org/apps/news/story.asp?NewsID=16037andCr=birdandCr1=flu]

[131] Reuters Foundation, "ETHIOPIA: Birds Test Negative for avian flu." December 20, 2005. [http://www.alertnet.org]

[132] SAID, *H5N1 Avian Influenza (AI) Most Recent Developments and Actions.* November 26 - December 19, 2005.

[133] Grudgings, Stuart, "Rich-poor divide hoblles Asia's bird flu plans." Reuters, September 13, 2005. [http://www.reuters.com]

[134] GovEXEC.com, "House panel calls plan for tracking avian influenza 'inadequate'." December 7, 2005. [http://govexec.com/dailyfed/1205/120705cdpm2.htm]

[135] Grudgings, Stuart, "Rich-poor divide hobbles Asia's bird flu plans." Reuters. September 13, 2005. [http://www.reuters.com]

[136] ASEAN Plus Three consists of the ASEAN countries plus China, Japan, and South Korea.

[137] Participants in the first EAS included the ten ASEAN members (Brunei, Burma, Cambodia, Indonesia, Laos, Malaysia, Philippines, Singapore, Thailand, and Vietnam), the "plus three" states (China, South Korea, and Japan), as well as Australia, New Zealand, and India. For more on the summit, see CRS Report RS22346, *East Asian Summit: Issues for Congress*, by Bruce Vaughn.

[138] Ilaria Capua and Stafano Manganon, "Vaccination for Avian Influenza in Asia," *Vaccine*, Vol. 22, 2004, pp. 4137-4138.

[139] Perry, Michael, "Poor Asian farmers are weak link in bird flu fight." Reuters. September 19, 2005. [http://www.alertnet.org/thenews/newsdesk/SYD28137.htm]

[140] World Bank, "New Global Program to Deal with Avian Flu." November 4, 2005. [http://www.worldbank.org]

[141] ADB, "ADB Support for Asia's Fight Against Avian Flu Could Reach $470 Million." November 9, 2005. [http://www.adb.org/Documents/News/2005/nr2005173.asp]

[142] Osterholm, Michael, "Preparing for the Next Pandemic." Foreign Affairs, July/August 2005. [http://www.foreignaffairs.org].

[143] Ibid. Country-specific SARS-related information, including costs and fatalities can be found in CRS Report RL32072, *Severe Acute Respiratory Syndrome (SARS): The International Response*, by Rhoda Margesson and Tiaji Salaam.

[144] Nordland, Rod and George Wehrfritz, "A Costly Disease: Europe and the rest of the world braces for the economic fallout of a possible bird-

flu pandemic." October 24, 2005. [http://msnbc.msn.com/id/9711926/site/newsweek/]
[145] World Bank East Asia and Pacific Region, "Spread of Avian Flu Could Affect Next Year's Economic Outlook." November 2005. [http://siteresources.worldbank.org/INTEAPHALFYEARLYUPDATE/Resources/EAP-Brief-avian-flu.pdf]
[146] U.S. Trade Representative Robert Portman discussion at the US-ASEAN Business Council Second Annual Asia Forum, November 1, 2005.
[147] USTR website, "America's Trade with China." April 21, 2004. [http://www.ustr.gov]
[148] USTR website, "Real Results in U.S. Trade with China." September 9, 2004. [http://www.ustr.gov]
[149] Bullion, Alan, "Threats on the Wing." The World Today, August/September 2005. Also see, Bradsher, Keith, "Some Asian Bankers Worry About the Economic Toll From Bird Flu." New York Times. April 5, 2005. [http://www.nytimes.com]
[150] CBO, *A Potential Influenza Pandemic: Possible Macroeconomic Effects and Policy Issues.* December 8, 2005. [http://www.cbo.gov/ftpdocs/69xx/doc6946/12-08-BirdFlu.pdf]
[151] Kilman, Scott, "Vaccine Remains Sticking Point in U.S. Defense Against Bird Flu." December 12, 2005. [http://www.wsj.com]. Basic screening tests for bird flu used by many importing countries leave ambiguous whether a bird testing positive is infected with H5N1 or has been vaccinated against it.
[152] Kolata, Gina, "Experts Unlock Clues to Spread of 1918 Flu Virus." New York Times, October 6, 2005. [http://www.nytimes.com]
[153] Ibid.
[154] CDC, "Possession, Use, and Transfer of Select Agents and Toxins — Reconstructed Replication Competent Forms of the 1918 Pandemic Influenza Virus Containing Any Portion of the Coding Regions of All Eight Gene Segments." 70 Federal Register 61407, October 20, 2005.
[155] For more information, see the CDC Select Agent Program page at [http://www.cdc.gov/od/sap] and CRS Report RL31719, *An Overview of the U.S. Public Health System in the Context of Emergency Preparedness*, by Sarah A. Lister.
[156] Altman, Lawrence and Keith Bradsher, "Vaccine Alone Won't Stem Avian Flu, Experts Warn." New York Times. August 8, 2005. [http://www.nytimes.com]
[157] Interview with State Department staff, October 18, 2005.

[158] Abbott, Alison, "The flu HQ." Nature, Volume 414, November 1, 2001. [http://www.nature.com]

In: Global Spread of the Avian Flu… ISBN 1-60021-011-2
Editors: M.R. Bethe, pp. 59-67

Chapter 2

AVIAN INFLUENZA: AGRICULTURAL ISSUES*

Jim Monke

SUMMARY

Since the fall of 2003, a strain of highly pathogenic avian influenza (H5N1) has spread throughout Asia, infecting mostly poultry but also a limited number of humans. In recent months, the virus has spread into parts of Europe. Controlling avian flu in poultry is seen as the best way to prevent a human pandemic from developing, by reducing the number of animal hosts in which the virus may evolve.

Avian flu can be highly contagious in domestic poultry. Strict biosecurity measures are practiced among commercial poultry farms and are encouraged by governments. The economic effects of any avian influenza outbreak can be significant, especially given international trade restrictions. This report will be updated as events warrant.

* Excerpted from CRS Report RS21747, dated November 10, 2005.

Status of Avian Influenza Outbreaks

In the United States

The highly pathogenic H5N1 strain of current global concern has not reached the United States, neither in poultry nor humans. (This report primarily addresses avian flu in poultry, although some human dimensions are discussed.) The most recent cases in domestic poultry were in 2004, with three unrelated and less pathogenic strains.

To reduce the possibility that H5N1 enters U.S. borders, the U.S. Department of Agriculture (USDA) has blocked imports of poultry and poultry products from affected countries. The Department of Homeland Security helps with enforcement through Customs and Border Protection. Surveillance of migratory birds is increasing.[1]

In the Rest of the World

Since December 2003, as many as nine Asian countries have had confirmed outbreaks or instances of H5N1 in poultry, including Vietnam, Thailand, Indonesia, Cambodia, China and Hong Kong, South Korea, Malaysia, Laos, and Japan. More recently, in the summer and fall of 2005, H5N1 spread westward and has been confirmed in at least five new countries: Russia, Kazakhstan, Turkey, Romania, and Croatia. Wild birds seem to be one of the main carriers, but their role in spreading the virus is not completely understood. The risk and likelihood of the virus spreading into Africa and the Middle East is increasing. Other countries on migratory bird routes are increasing surveillance efforts.

As the virus spreads, and becomes endemic in countries with low levels of veterinary services or animal husbandry practices that harbor the virus, the chances increase that the virus will evolve through mutation or reassortment into a strain that could be transmitted easily between humans. Thus, many experts call for the swift and coordinated control of avian flu in poultry as the best way to prevent a human pandemic from developing, by reducing the number of animal hosts in which the virus may evolve.[2]

The situation in Asia is historically unprecedented and extremely challenging. The United Nations Food and Agriculture Organization (FAO) estimates that over 130 million birds have died or been culled in Asia. Some countries were reluctant to acknowledge the disease for fear of economic consequences. In other countries, lack of compensation for farmers whose flocks are destroyed has been a disincentive to report outbreaks early. In some parts of Asia, about 80% of the poultry are produced in small backyard farms scattered throughout rural areas, further complicating control.

Two Forms with Many Strains

Avian influenza (AI) viruses exist throughout the world in many different strains. Avian flu is an Influenza A virus that infects birds, and certain strains have been known to infect both animals and humans. Avian flu is characterized by two forms in birds:

- a low pathogenicity (LPAI) form that causes mild illness, and
- a highly pathogenic (HPAI) form that is extremely contagious, causes severe illness, and frequently has high rates of mortality.[3]

Both forms are possible in several strains. Strains are identified by two surface proteins designated by the letters H and N.[4] Some low pathogenic strains (H5 and H7) are capable of mutating into highly pathogenic strains, and are thus treated nearly as aggressively. For example, during a 1999-2001 epidemic in Italy, an LPAI virus (H7N1) mutated into HPAI within nine months.

Because LPAI is endemic in wild bird populations, low pathogenicity outbreaks are not uncommon. The 2004 outbreaks in the United States included low pathogenicity strains of H7N2 in Delaware, Maryland, and New Jersey, and H2N2 in Pennsylvania. A strain classified as highly pathogenic H5N2 was found in Texas, although it did not manifest as highly pathogenic. Other recent outbreaks in U.S. poultry include low pathogenicity H7N2 in Connecticut and Rhode Island in 2003, and in Virginia, West Virginia, and North Carolina in 2002. There have been only three highly pathogenic outbreaks in the United States (1924, 1983, and 2004).

Transmission

Wild birds are the primary natural reservoir for Influenza A viruses and are often the vector that introduces new outbreaks into domestic flocks. Wild birds often are resistant to the virus and do not show clinical symptoms. The role of migratory birds is of increasing concern, although, in the past, scientists have not been sure that infected birds were able to migrate long distances.

Avian flu can be highly contagious in domestic poultry. The virus is spread by contact with infected feces, nasal, or eye excretions. Once present in domestic flocks, human activity becomes a risk for further transmission as people, clothing, vehicles, and supplies move between farms. Thus, strict biosecurity measures are practiced among commercial poultry farms and are encouraged by USDA and international agricultural organizations such as the FAO.[5]

In the United States, avian flu viruses have been common in live bird markets concentrated in urban areas with ethnic communities. Biosecurity practices can often be lacking or insufficient if birds and equipment intermingle in the market or move back to farms. Thus sanitation of crates, periodic disinfection of the market, and restrictions on moving birds back into general farm populations are needed. USDA has focused on these markets as one of the first places to control the disease. Live bird markets are a small portion of the U.S. poultry industry (about 1/4 of 1%), but the frequency of outbreaks is of concern to the majority of commercial growers practicing tighter biosecurity protocols. In Asia, a larger network of live bird markets and the much larger number of small backyard farms have posed significant problems for eradicating the disease.

Human Infection

Avian flu can infect humans through poultry-to-human transmission, usually through contact with fecal matter or other live bird excretions. The World Health Organization (WHO) and the World Organization for Animal Health (OIE) conclude that avian flu is not a food-borne disease since the virus is killed by the temperature reached in normal cooking. The Centers for Disease Control and Prevention (CDC) recommends standard food safety practices.

The human disease caused by H5N1 differs from typical human flu. H5N1 can replicate in a wide range of cells, more so than the usual flu virus. This can result in a severe disseminated disease affecting multiple organs, which has caused high rates of mortality. The human vaccine currently available for mass inoculation in the fall of 2005 is felt to offer little protection against H5N1; vaccine trials and development are underway. Public health professionals are concerned that the virus could mutate or combine with human flu viruses. If such a mutation were to occur, allowing efficient human-to-human transmission, a more serious public health problem would result.

The number of human cases of H5N1 confirmed by WHO during the current outbreak (December 2003-November 9, 2005) totals 125, resulting in 64 deaths (a 51% mortality rate). Four countries have had human cases: Vietnam (92 cases, 42 deaths), Thailand (20 cases, 13 deaths), Indonesia (9 cases, 5 deaths), and Cambodia (4 cases and 4 deaths). Some scientists believe that if the virus evolves to allow human-to-human transmission, the mortality rate may decline, but whether this happens remains unknown.

The first human cases of H5N1 were in Hong Kong in 1997 (18 cases, 6 deaths). Two other strains are documented to cause human illness: H7N7 in the Netherlands in 2003 (83 cases, 1 death), and H9N2 in Hong Kong in 1999 and 2003 (3 cases).

In the United States, the 2002 low pathogenic outbreak in poultry in Virginia resulted in limited evidence of one human case. A man involved in the poultry depopulation effort was found to have antibodies for H7N2 avian flu. In the fall of 2003, a man from Westchester County, New York, contracted and recovered from H7N2 avian flu. The case was not initially diagnosed as avian flu, and CDC first confirmed diagnosis in April 2004.

CONTROL

Controlling avian flu in poultry through prevention and eradication is done domestically by individual farmers in cooperation with state and federal governments, and with industry associations and international organizations. In the United States, the USDA Animal and Plant Health Inspection Service (APHIS) is the lead federal agency.

Internationally, the U.N. Food and Agriculture Organization (FAO) has a joint response plan with WHO for the current outbreak. The $140 million, three-year plan is being implemented but is not fully funded by donor countries. The United States has contributed about $25 million.[6]

Preventing Infection

Biosecurity practices are the most important means of preventing outbreaks in poultry. This includes preventing access of wild birds to domestic flocks and limiting access to farm buildings by outside conveyances. For example, delivery trucks and personnel are cleaned and disinfected before entering a farm's biosecure area. In Asia and other parts of the world, the large number of small farms or backyard flocks without biosecurity practices has posed greater problems for control. Such animal husbandry practices are slow to change.

Eradicating Outbreaks

Because the virus is highly contagious and easily spread in poultry, the most common method of control after there is an outbreak is culling (also called "stamping out," depopulating) the infected flocks, and certain flocks in close proximity to the infected flock. Federal statute allows such destruction of animals (9 CFR 53.4). Quarantines of surrounding areas are imposed (usually by state authorities) until the disease is eradicated. Following depopulation, buildings and equipment are rigorously disinfected before new birds are allowed, a process that takes at least several weeks. The virus is killed by common disinfectants or heat (about 160 degrees F).

Vaccines

While vaccination of poultry is possible and has been used on a small scale with some success, it generally is not considered a viable or sufficient control method. Vaccination poses problems for international trade as many countries will not import Poultry products from other countries that use vaccination as a means of control, since animals will test positive for antibodies. If vaccination is not administered and monitored correctly, it can also allow the virus to become endemic and continue to spread or mutate.[7]

In November 2005, USDA has a stockpile of 40 million doses of vaccine (for two types of H5 and two types of H7 viruses). The Administration's recent funding request for avian flu (discussed below) includes a proposal to double USDA's stockpile.

Federal Response to Domestic Outbreaks

Domestic outbreaks usually are managed through joint federal, state, and industry cooperation. States usually lead the response in terms of depopulation and quarantines. APHIS provides personnel and equipment to advise and supplement state resources. In highly pathogenic outbreaks, APHIS may take a larger role. The USDA National Veterinary Services Lab (NVSL) in Ames, IA, conducts confirmatory tests on the pathogenicity and type of virus. USDA also works to limit export restrictions to small geographic areas (such as states or counties) and reopen export markets once outbreaks are eradicated.

Indemnities to Farmers

Compensation programs are desired to encourage farmers to report outbreaks and cooperate with disease control programs. Indemnification programs for low pathogenicity outbreaks generally are managed by the states. Some industry associations, such as those on the Delmarva peninsula (Delaware, Maryland, and Virginia), have compensation funds. In the past, USDA has not had a standing compensation program for low pathogenicity avian influenza.[8] However, a new program is being developed following increased appropriations for a low pathogenicity program in FY2005. When indemnification is offered by USDA, the standard rate for low pathogenicity programs is 50% of fair market value. For highly pathogenic outbreaks of avian flu, statute allows USDA to offer 100% indemnification (9 CFR 53.2).

ECONOMIC IMPACTS

The economic effects of any avian influenza outbreak can be significant. Expenses to conduct depopulation and quarantines, as well as the direct loss of production, affect local farms and regions. However, bigger economic effects come from international trade bans. Localized quarantines and bans on the sale or movement of birds can affect farmers outside the immediate quarantine area.

The United States is the world's largest producer and exporter of poultry meat and the second-largest egg producer. USDA estimates that about 8.5 billion broilers were produced in 2003, and total poultry production was worth $23.3 billion (out of $105 billion for all livestock, and $200 billion total of crops and livestock). Broiler production was valued at $15.2 billion, followed by eggs at $5.3 billion, and turkeys at $2.7 billion. The U.S. exports about 16% of its poultry production.[9]

No estimates of the potential effect from an H5N1 outbreak in the United States are available because of the highly uncertain nature of any possible, hypothetical outbreak. The 1983-84 outbreak of highly pathogenic avian flu in the United States caused the destruction of 17 million birds and cost $65 million. In the small 2004 domestic outbreak, about 400,000 chickens were depopulated in the United States. This was less than 1/200 of 1% of the 8.5 billion broilers slaughtered in the U.S. for food annually. Yet, the effect on local regions and individual farms can was much greater.

Federal Appropriations to Control Avian Flu in Poultry

Federal appropriations for avian influenza have grown significantly in recent years. In FY2004, Congress provided APHIS with $994,000 for avian flu for monitoring and control. Following the 2004 domestic outbreak, USDA used emergency authority to release $13.7 million of Commodity Credit Corporation (CCC) funds to accelerate its avian flu plans. In FY2005, Congress appropriated APHIS $23.8 million for avian flu, with about half for indemnities. For FY2006, the APHIS appropriation for avian flu is $13.8 million. The conference agreement for agriculture appropriations (H.R. 2744, H.Rept. 109-255) notes that $28.3 million is available, including carryover, with about $12 million for indemnities.

The Emergency Supplemental Appropriations Act of 2005 (P.L. 109-13) provided $25 million to the U.S. Agency for International Development (USAID) and CDC to combat the spread of avian flu. Conferees encourage U.S. cooperation to support FAO and WHO on a joint international plan (the FAO/WHO plan mentioned above).

On November 1, 2005, President Bush submitted a request to Congress for $7.1 billion in emergency funding to address avian flu in both humans and poultry. Of this amount, $91 million would go to USDA ($73 million to APHIS for domestic activities, $7 million to the Agricultural Research Service, and $11 million for international activities in the form of technical assistance on surveillance, biosecurity, culling, vaccination, and control).

Reference

[1] For domestic issues related to avian flu in poultry, see the U.S. Department of Agriculture (USDA) at [http://www.aphis.usda.gov/lpa/issues/avian_influenza]. For background on human issues, see the Centers for Disease Control (CDC) at [http://www.cdc.gov/flu/avian].

[2] International organizations include the U.N. Food and Agriculture Organization (FAO) [http://www.fao.org/ag/againfo/subjects/en/health/diseases-cards/special_avian.html], the World Health Organization (WHO) [http://www.who.int/csr/disease/avian_influenza/en], and the World Organization for Animal Health (OIE) [http://www.oie.int/eng/avian_influenza].

[3] Tests for pathogenicity are conducted in two ways. The first is through genetic (DNA) sequencing. The other is by inoculating healthy chickens and monitoring their immune response and mortality over a 10-day period. HPAI strains can result in greater or lesser rates of mortality, perhaps ranging from 30-100%. LPAI strains typically do not exceed 10-20 percent mortality.

[4] The surface proteins are called hemagglutinin and neuraminidase, abbreviated H and N. Fifteen H subtypes and nine N subtypes have been identified, and they can occur in any combination.

[5] For biosecurity recommendations, see the USDA "Biosecurity for the Birds" website at [http://www.aphis.usda.gov/vs/birdbiosecurity/hpai.html].

[6] "A Global Strategy for the Progressive Control of Highly Pathogenic Avian Influenza (HPAI)," U.N. Food and Agriculture Organization (FAO) and World Organization for Animal Health (OIE), in cooperation with the World Health Organization (WHO), November 2005 [http://www.fao.org/ag/againfo/subjects/documents/ai/HPAIGlobalStrategy31Oct05.pdf].

[7] See two journal articles by scientists at the World Organization for Animal Health (OIE): Ilaria Capua and Stephano Marangon, "Vaccination for avian influenza in Asia," *Vaccine*, 22 (2004), 4137-7138 [http://www.oie.int/eng/avian_influenza/vaccination%20in%20Asia.pdf], and Ilaria Capua and Stephano Marangon, "The use of vaccination as an option for the control of avian influenza," Technical Item of the 71st General Session of the OIE, May 2003, [http://www.oie.int/eng/avian_influenza/A_71%20SG_12_CS3E.pdf].

[8] A limited USDA indemnification program was created for an LPAI outbreak in Virginia in 2002 (9 CFR 53.11). The Administration's FY2005 budget request includes a proposal for an LPAI indemnification program.

[9] The top five states in broiler production are Georgia (15%), Arkansas (14%), Alabama (13%), Mississippi (9%), and North Carolina (9%), totaling 60% of U.S. broiler production.

In: Global Spread of the Avian Flu... ISBN 1-60021-011-2
Editors: M.R. Bethe, pp. 69-78

Chapter 3

AVIAN INFLUENZA: MULTIPLE STRAINS CAUSE DIFFERENT EFFECTS WORLDWIDE*

Jim Monke

SUMMARY

Since the fall of 2003, highly pathogenic avian influenza (H5N1) has spread throughout Asia, infecting mostly poultry but also a limited number of humans. Officials are concerned that the virus could mutate to allow human-to-human transmission. The situation in Asia has raised the awareness of this disease in the U.S.

In February and March 2004, a low pathogenicity avian flu surfaced in Delaware, Maryland, and New Jersey (H7N2), and another strain was found in Pennsylvania (H2N2). One highly pathogenic strain (H5N2) surfaced in Texas. In British Columbia, Canada, a highly pathogenic strain (H7N3) was discovered in March, and an H5 strain was found in May. While low pathogenicity avian flu (LPAI) is not uncommon, the strain in Texas is the first highly pathogenic (HPAI) case in the U.S. since 1983-1984. Federal and state officials have responded by depopulating (destroying) flocks, imposing quarantines, conducting extensive surveillance, and providing funding.

---

* Excerpted from CRS Report RS21747, dated May 14, 2004.

On April 1, USDA announced that the HPAI outbreak in Texas was eradicated. In Canada, however, the disease has spread extensively and depopulation is underway.

Only a few strains of avian flu have been known to affect humans, and no humans in the U.S. have been known to be infected. In Canada, however, two workers in the response were infected and have recovered. Because human infection is possible, public health guidelines have been published. This report will be updated as events warrant.

TYPES OF AVIAN INFLUENZA

Many different strains of avian influenza (avian flu) virus exist throughout the world. Avian flu is a form of the Influenza A virus that infects birds, and certain strains have been known to infect both animals and humans.[1] The Centers for Disease Control and Prevention (CDC) notes that avian flu viruses rarely infect humans, but recommends that those involved in control efforts engage in activities to minimize their risks. Officials are concerned that the virus could mutate and cause a pandemic through human-to-human transmission. The Office International des Epizooties (OIE) and World Health Organization (WHO) conclude that poultry products from affected countries do not pose any human food safety risk, and CDC recommends standard food safety practices.[2]

Wild birds are the primary natural reservoir for Influenza A and are often the vector that introduces new outbreaks into domestic flocks. The virus can be highly contagious in domestic poultry, which are not as resistant as wild birds. Avian flu is spread by contact with infected feces, nasal or eye excretions, or equipment, vehicles, or clothes. Once present in domestic flocks, human activity becomes a risk for further transmission.

The virus has been common in live bird markets concentrated in urban areas with ethnic communities. The U.S. Department of Agriculture (USDA) has focused on these markets as one of the first places to control the disease. Live bird markets are a small portion of the U.S. poultry industry (about 1/4 of 1%), but the frequency of outbreaks is of concern to the majority of commercial growers practicing tighter biosecurity protocols.

Two Forms with Many Strains

Avian influenza has two forms in birds: a low pathogenicity (LPAI) form that causes mild illness, and a highly pathogenic (HPAI) form that is extremely contagious, causes severe illness, and frequently has high rates of mortality. Both forms are possible in several strains. Strains are identified by two surface proteins designated by the letters H and N.[3] Some LPAI strains are capable of mutating into HPAI.[4] Thus, LPAI is treated nearly as aggressively as HPAI. LPAI is not required to be reported to the OIE, but USDA does report it to OIE as a practical matter.

In addition to the HPAI strains of H5N1 in Asia, H5N2 in Texas, and H7N3 in British Columbia, other recent occurrences of HPAI include Hong Kong in 1997, and the Netherlands in 2003. Before 2004, the last U.S. outbreak of HPAI was in 1983-84, when cases of H5N2 caused the destruction of 17 million birds and cost $65 million.

Because LPAI is endemic in wild bird populations, outbreaks are not uncommon. In addition to the current LPAI strains of H7N2 and H2N2 in U.S., other recent LPAI outbreaks in U.S. poultry include H7N2 in Connecticut and Rhode Island during 2003, and in Virginia, West Virginia, and North Carolina in 2002.[5]

Because the virus is highly contagious and easily spread, the most common method of control is culling (depopulation, or killing) the infected flocks,[6] and quarantine of affected areas until the disease is no longer present. While vaccination is possible and has been tested on a small scale, it is not widely considered a viable control method.[7] After the contaminated flock is depopulated, buildings and equipment are rigorously disinfected before new birds are allowed, a process that takes at least several weeks. The virus is killed by common disinfectants or heat (about 70 degrees C, or 160 degrees F).

Avian Flu in the United States

In February and March 2004, a number of LPAI outbreaks occurred in Delaware, Maryland, Pennsylvania and New Jersey, and an HPAI strain was found in Texas. These outbreaks are unrelated to the H5N1 virus in Asia.

LPAI

On February 6, 2004, a flock of 12,000 chickens in Kent County, Delaware, tested positive for H7N2. The flock was destroyed and composted. On February 10, 2004, a commercial flock tested positive for the same strain about 5 miles from the first outbreak. Delaware depopulated that 73,800-chicken flock, temporarily banned live poultry sales, and expanded the quarantine to about 80 farms in a six mile radius. On February 12, four live bird markets in New Jersey were discovered with the same H7N2 strain, and a link was found to the first case in Delaware. Also on February 12, a flock in Lancaster County, Pennsylvania, tested positive for H2N2. Later, on March 5, a commercial flock of about 330,000 chickens in Pocomoke City, Maryland, tested positive for H7N2 and was subsequently destroyed.

All subsequent tests of farms in Delaware, Maryland, and Pennsylvania have been negative for the disease. At least 1,736 farms and 4,242 chicken houses have been tested (counting initial and repeated tests), and all had negative results. Background testing continues and flocks going to slaughter receive pre-movement avian flu testing.

HPAI

On February 17, a flock of 6,600 chickens in Gonzales County, Texas, was found to be positive for an H5 strain of avian flu. The flock was depopulated on February 21. The same strain was also found in two live bird markets in Houston, and those birds were depopulated along with birds at three other Houston live bird markets. USDA tests confirm that the strain is H5N2 and genetic indicators suggested that the virus was highly pathogenic by OIE standards.[8] USDA activated its response system and established an incident command post in Texas. Five rounds of surveillance testing followed and all had negative results. The quarantine was lifted March 29 and the command post closed. On April 1, USDA notified OIE that the HPAI outbreak was eradicated. Routine surveillance will continue until mid June. No commercial poultry flocks were infected in Texas.

Federal Response

In this recent U.S. outbreak, the disease has been managed through state-level responses in terms of depopulation and quarantines. USDA's

Animal and Plant Health Inspection Service (APHIS) provided personnel and equipment to advise and supplement state resources. For the HPAI strain in Texas, USDA set up an incident response center on site. The USDA National Veterinary Services Lab (NVSL) in Ames, IA, conducted confirmatory tests on the pathogenicity and type of virus for all cases.

USDA also is working to reopen export markets in countries that have banned poultry imports from the U.S. or certain states. Reopening trade in LPAI cases is easier than under HPAI cases. Generally, once a third confirmation test for LPAI is completed (about two weeks after the initial outbreak) and no further cases are found, negotiations to reopen trade can be resumed. Similar eradication efforts are undertaken for HPAI, but importing countries often are more reluctant to lift trade restrictions. USDA is working to preserve exports for states and regions not infected with avian flu by encouraging countries to limit their bans to affected areas rather than the entire United States.

AVIAN FLU IN CANADA

On March 9, Canada discovered avian flu in southern British Columbia. The highly pathogenic H7N3 virus has since spread throughout the Fraser Valley area. The Canadian government initially depopulated 9,000 birds, and then another 275,000 birds on March 24. But the virus continued to spread and, as of May 12, has been confirmed on 40 farms. On April 5, the Minister of Agriculture announced the depopulation of all commercial and backyard poultry flocks in the Fraser Valley "control area." Approximately 19 million birds will be destroyed, although non-infected flocks can be sold under certain conditions. Unlike in the U.S., where birds were composted on site, Canada is trucking carcasses to incinerators or landfills, and this poses additional risks for spreading the virus. The U.S. has increased surveillance in Washington state, placed a ban on live poultry imports from British Columbia, and tightened restrictions for poultry products. Although no new H7 cases have been found since April 29, an H5 virus was discovered on a Fraser Valley farm on May 11. Further genetic tests will confirm the strain and pathogenicity.

AVIAN FLU IN ASIA

As of April 1, 2004, 10 Asian countries have reported current outbreaks of HPAI. Nine countries have confirmed subtype H5N1, including Cambodia, China and Hong Kong, Indonesia, Japan, Laos, South Korea, Thailand, and Vietnam. Pakistan had an outbreak of HPAI H7. Though progress in controlling the virus is reported in some areas, Vietnam and Thailand have had small scale recurrences. The U.N. Food and Agriculture Organization (FAO) estimates that over 100 million birds have died or been culled. The United States has imposed trade restrictions.

The situation in Asia is historically unprecedented and extremely challenging. Some countries were reluctant to acknowledge the disease for fear of economic consequences.[9] In some of these countries, around 80% of the poultry are produced in small backyard farms scattered throughout rural areas, further complicating control.

HUMAN INFECTION

Avian flu can infect humans through poultry-to-human transmission, usually through contact with fecal matter or other live bird excretions. The first such transmission was in 1997 in Hong Kong with H5N1 (18 cases, 6 deaths). Two other strains have been documented to cause human illness: H7N7 in the Netherlands in 2003 (83 cases, 1 death), and H9N2 in Hong Kong in 1999 and 2003 (3 cases). The human disease caused by H5N1 differs from typical human flu. H5N1 can replicate in a wide range of cells, resulting in a severe disseminated disease affecting multiple organs and causing high rates of mortality. Public health professionals are concerned that the virus could mutate or combine with human flu viruses. If such a mutation were to occur, allowing efficient human-to-human transmission, a more serious public health problem would result. The human vaccine currently available is felt to offer little protection against this strain.

In the current outbreak, as of April 5, Thailand and Vietnam have reported 34 human cases of N5N1 infection, resulting in 24 deaths. In Canada, two humans who had separate exposure to infected birds tested positive for H7 infection. Both experienced mild symptoms and have fully recovered.

In the U.S., the 2002 outbreak in poultry in Virginia resulted in limited evidence of one human case. A man involved in the poultry depopulation effort was found to have antibodies for H7N2 avian flu. In the fall of 2003, a man from Westchester County, New York, contracted and recovered from H7N2 avian flu. The case was not initially believed to be avian flu, and CDC first confirmed the H7N2 diagnosis in April 2004. Officials have not determined how the man contracted the disease.

ECONOMIC EFFECTS

Indemnities to Farmers

The economic effects of any avian influenza outbreak can be significant, particularly given the standard depopulation method of control. So far in 2004, over 422,000 chickens have been depopulated in the U.S. as a result of avian influenza.[10] Localized quarantines and bans on the sale or movement of birds can affect farmers outside the immediate quarantine area in affected states.

Indemnification programs for LPAI generally are managed by the states. While USDA can offer indemnities to farmers whose flocks are destroyed due to HPAI, USDA does not have a standing indemnification program for LPAI.[11] When indemnification is offered by USDA, the standard rate is 50% of fair market value (FMV), but a 100% indemnification rate is allowed for HPAI (9 CFR 53.2).

Poultry Supply and Demand

In the mid-Atlantic region, Delaware, Maryland, Virginia, and Pennsylvania account for about 10% of U.S. broiler production. Texas accounts for about 7% of broiler production. Thus, while production in these areas is not insignificant, the affected states are not among the major poultry producing states in the U.S.[12] In areas affected by quarantines, non-infected flocks will eventually be marketed once officials determine that it is safe to transport the birds. Thus the overall supply of poultry to the U.S. market is not expected to decrease noticeably. In terms of domestic consumption, avian flu is not expected to reduce consumer confidence in poultry, given the steady demand for beef even after the discovery of BSE in the U.S. in December 2003. However, in Asia, anecdotal evidence suggests declining poultry supplies due to widespread Asian depopulation efforts is causing poultry prices to rise there.[13]

The U.S. exports about 16% of its poultry production. The largest importer is Russia, accounting for about 30% of poultry exports in 2003. Other primary importers of U.S poultry products include Mexico, Hong Kong, Canada and Japan. As of May 11, 50 foreign countries have imposed restrictions on importing U.S. poultry and poultry products. At this point, Canada has lifted its restrictions, and Russia and the European Union have only regional restrictions. However, Mexico, Japan, and South Korea, among others, have placed country-wide bans on U.S. poultry, affecting over 10% of such exports. USDA negotiates with each country regarding easing restrictions, especially after the disease is contained and assurances can provided for the safety of U.S. products.

Feed and Other Inputs

The outbreak of avian flu in Asia had an impact on U.S. exports of feed ingredients (especially soybeans and soybean meal) to the region. Yet despite the potential for lower exports of soybeans to Asia, soybean prices in the U.S. are at (or near) record highs because unusually low domestic supplies and strong domestic demand were already forecast to cause a shortage of soybeans during the summer of 2004. Thus, avian flu is not expected to significantly affect U.S. soybean prices since the tight domestic market situation is of greater magnitude.

Federal Appropriations to Control Avian Flu in Poultry

For FY2004, Congress appropriated APHIS $994,000 for avian flu (primarily for control in live bird markets), and the Agricultural Research Service (ARS) $2 million for research. On May 12, 2004, USDA released $13.7 million of Commodity Credit Corporation (CCC) funds to begin a larger, national LPAI program ($10.8 million) and assist Texas with the HPAI outbreak ($2.9 million). This CCC transfer effectively accelerates the APHIS plan to increase its avian flu program, as described below.

For FY2005, APHIS requested a significant increase to expand its avian flu program from $1 million to $12.7 million. This is a rare increase in the

FY2005 APHIS pest and disease management function, which otherwise is flat or shrinking in the Administration's proposal. About half of the funding would be used for indemnities when flocks are destroyed. Other initiatives include cooperative agreements with states, increased monitoring, a bird identification system, laboratory support, and vaccine development. ARS requests $2 million for avian flu research in FY2005. A "Dear Colleague" letter by Representatives Etheridge and Pickering began circulating in the House at the end of March requesting $25 million for avian flu at APHIS in FY2005.

REFERENCES

[1] The primary focus of this report is the effect on agriculture.

[2] For more information about avian flu, please see the U.S. Department of Agriculture (USDA) at [http://www.aphis.usda.gov/lpa/issues /ai_us/ai_us.html], the World Health Organization (WHO) at [http://www.who.int/csr/disease/avian_influenza/en/], the Centers for Disease Control (CDC) at [http://www.cdc.gov/flu/avian/index.htm], and the Office International des Epizooties (OIE) at [http://www.oie.int/eng/avian_influenza/home.htm]. The United Nations Food and Agriculture Organization (FAO) website also includes several maps showing the situation in Asia at [http://www.fao.org/ag/againfo/subjects/en/health/diseases-cards/special_avian.html].

[3] The surface proteins are called hemagglutinin and neuraminidase, abbreviated H and N. Fifteen H subtypes and nine N subtypes have been identified, and they can occur in any combination.

[4] For example, during a 1999-2001 epidemic in Italy, an LPAI virus (H7N1) mutated into HPAI within nine months. More than 13 million birds died or were destroyed.

[5] For a more complete list, see USDA at [http://www.aphis.usda.gov /lpa/issues/ai_us/ai_us.html].

[6] See 9 CFR 53.4, "Destruction of animals."

[7] Ilaria Capua and Stafano Marangon. "The Use of Vaccination as an Option for the Control of Avian Influenza," OIE International Committee 71st General Session, May 18-23, 2003, at [http://www.oie.int/downld/71SG_2003/A_71%20SG_12_CS3E.pdf].

[8] Test for pathogenicity are conducted in two ways. The first is through genetic (DNA) sequencing. The other is by inoculating healthy

chickens and monitoring their immune response and mortality over a 10-day period. HPAI strains can result in greater or lesser rates of mortality, perhaps ranging from 30-100%. LPAI strains typically do not exceed 10-20 percent mortality.

[9] For more about the political impact of avian flu in China, see CRS Report RL32227, *SARS, Avian Flu, and Other Challenges for China's Political, Social, and Economic Transformation.*

[10] For perspective, 8.5 billion broilers were slaughtered for food in the U.S. in 2003. The current depopulation statistic is about 1/200 of 1% of that annual slaughter number.

[11] A limited USDA indemnification program was created for an LPAI outbreak in Virginia in 2002 (9 CFR 53.11). The Administration's FY2005 budget request includes a proposal for an LPAI indemnification program.

[12] The top five states in broiler production are Georgia (15%), Arkansas (14%), Alabama (13%), Mississippi (9%), and North Carolina (9%), totaling 60% of U.S. broiler production.

[13] World Perspectives, Inc. "Ag Perspectives," February 20, 2004.

In: Global Spread of the Avian Flu... ISBN 1-60021-011-2
Editors: M.R. Bethe, pp. 79-120

Chapter 4

PANDEMIC INFLUENZA: DOMESTIC PREPAREDNESS EFFORTS*

Sarah A. Lister

SUMMARY

In 1997, a new avian influenza virus (H5N1 avian flu) emerged in Hong Kong, killing six people. This was the first time that an avian influenza virus was shown to be transmitted directly from birds to humans. The virus persisted in the region, and has since spread to a number of Asian and European countries, where it has infected more than 120 people, killing more than 60. The severity of this strain is similar to that of the deadly 1918 Spanish flu, which caused a global pandemic that may have killed up to 2% of the world's population. Though influenza pandemics occur with some regularity, and the United States has been involved in specific planning efforts since the early 1990s, the H5N1 situation has created a sense of urgency among the world's public health officials.

Global pandemic preparedness and response efforts are coordinated by the World Health Organization (WHO). The U.S. Department of Health and Human Services (HHS) released a draft pandemic flu preparedness and response plan in August 2004, and a final plan in November 2005. President Bush announced a national

---

* Excerpted from CRS Report RL33145, dated November 10, 2005.

strategy to coordinate pandemic preparedness and response activities across federal agencies. Domestic response activities will be carried out under the broad, all-hazards blueprint for a coordinated federal, state and local response laid out in the National Response Plan, released by the Department of Homeland Security (DHS) in 2004.

Even in light of the plans discussed above, if a flu pandemic were to occur in the next several years, the U.S. response would be affected by the limited availability of a vaccine (the best preventive measure for flu), as well as by limited availability of certain drugs used to treat severe flu infections, and by the general lack of surge capacity within our healthcare system. The U.S. healthcare system is largely private, while the public health system is largely based in state, rather than federal, authority. This structure creates numerous challenges in assuring the needed response capacity, and coordinating the various response elements. Planning is further complicated by the fact that while periodic influenza pandemics have been seen over the years, their timing and severity have been unpredictable. This report will be updated to reflect changing circumstances.

INTRODUCTION

In 1997 a new strain of influenza (flu) jumped from poultry directly to humans in Hong Kong, causing several human deaths. This was the first documented occurrence of direct transmission of an avian flu virus from birds to people. Despite efforts to contain the virus through mass culling of poultry flocks, the virus (also called H5N1 for specific proteins on its surface) re-emerged in 2003. It has since been reported in domestic poultry and/or migratory birds in more than a dozen Asian countries, and in Europe.[1] Also since 2003, it has infected more than 120 people in Cambodia, Indonesia, Thailand, and Vietnam, resulting in more than 60 deaths.[2] As of yet the virus has not developed the ability to transmit efficiently from person to person. Were that to occur, a global influenza pandemic would be likely.

The high lethality of the H5N1 strain and its tendency to affect healthy young people remind health authorities of the deadly 1918 Spanish flu, which is estimated to have killed up to 2% of the world's population, and was a substantial cause of mortality in U.S. military personnel in World War I. The World Health Organization (WHO) says, "If an influenza pandemic virus were to appear again similar to the one that struck in 1918, even taking into account the advances in medicine since then, unparalleled tolls of illness and death could be expected."[3]

U.S. and world health authorities believe that while periodic influenza pandemics are inevitable, their progress may be slowed, and their impacts blunted, by rapid detection and local control efforts. The added time would allow affected countries to better manage the situation, and countries not yet affected to better prepare. To realize these benefits, countries affected by avian flu must be able to track the spread of the virus in birds, and quickly detect and investigate suspected human cases. Hence, a country's capabilities in epidemiology, laboratory detection and other public health services affect the welfare of the global community as well as the country itself. This fact presents developed nations with novel policy challenges, such as whether to reserve scarce health resources such as antiviral drugs for themselves, or to deploy them to other countries at the center of an emerging pandemic.

WHO released a pandemic preparedness plan in early 2005, updated from its prior 1999 draft. The United States released a draft pandemic plan in August 2004, a national strategy on November 1, 2005, and a final plan on November 2, 2005. States were required to prepare pandemic plans as a condition of their federal bioterrorism preparedness grants. The sudden shortage of seasonal flu vaccine in the United States for the 2004-2005 season offered an unplanned mini-drill for pandemic preparedness, highlighting the implications of limited vaccine and antiviral production capacity and the absence of a coordinated federal/state/local/private distribution system for vaccine distribution. In a pandemic, vaccine would likely be federally owned and distributed through a national system designed to support the Strategic National Stockpile. But antiviral drugs would be controlled by a mix of federal, state, local and private holders, and its distribution would likely face the same challenges posed by the 2004 seasonal flu vaccine shortage.

A recurring theme in WHO planning documents and consultations is the need for countries to engage sectors beyond healthcare and public health in preparedness and response. On October 27, 2005, Health and Human Services (HHS) Secretary Michael Leavitt said, "If a pandemic hits our shores, it will affect almost every sector of our society, not just health care, but transportation systems, workplaces, schools, public safety and more. It will require a coordinated government-wide response, including federal, state and local governments, and it will require the private sector and all of us as individuals to be ready."[4] A 1918-style pandemic could be so severe that non-health-related essential services would be impaired by high absenteeism or supply chain disruptions, and health services could be in such short supply that law enforcement protection might be required for them. Countries might seal their borders or take similar measures with impacts on trade and commerce, though WHO does not recommend this, except in some narrow circumstances for pre-pandemic control.

The HHS pandemic plan presumes that the National Response Plan would be activated, if needed, to streamline the federal response to a pandemic. Pandemic flu is different from most other types of emergencies (e.g., bombings or chemical attacks). Since flu is communicable, there is no discrete "scene" to secure, and all states might be affected nearly simultaneously.

The WHO stresses that the impact of an influenza pandemic would be greatest in developing countries, which lack vaccine production capacity, have limited means to purchase vaccines or antiviral drugs, and have more rudimentary public health and healthcare systems. The WHO notes that certain international efforts that help these nations respond to pandemics could help in other ways, too. For example, boosting demand for seasonal flu vaccine would boost global vaccine capacity. Also, investments in epidemiology and lab capacity for influenza would enhance capacity for disease control generally.

This report discusses pandemic influenza in general, previous pandemics and their global and domestic impacts, and the possible impacts of another pandemic caused by the H5N1 avian flu strain. It also discusses WHO and HHS preparedness plans and their context in broader emergency preparedness efforts. Finally, the report looks at a number of policy issues in pandemic influenza preparedness and response. While reference is made when relevant to global preparedness efforts and to animal health impacts, the focus of this report is U.S. domestic preparedness and response planning, and the projected impacts of an influenza pandemic on American citizens. For more information on seasonal influenza, vaccine development and shortages, see CRS Report RL32655, *Influenza Vaccine Shortages and Implications*, by Sarah A. Lister and Erin D. Williams. For more information on agricultural implications of avian flu, see CRS Report RS21747, *Avian Influenza: Agricultural Issues*, by Jim Monke. For more information the health response to disasters in general, see CRS Report RL33096, *2005 Gulf Coast Hurricanes: The Public Health and Medical Response*, by Sarah A. Lister. This report will be updated to reflect changing circumstances.

UNDERSTANDING PANDEMIC INFLUENZA

What is Pandemic Influenza?

A *pandemic* (from the Greek, for "all of the people") is an epidemic of human disease occurring over a very wide area, crossing international boundaries and affecting a large number of people. Though it does so with some regularity, influenza is not the only pathogen that causes pandemics. A pandemic of the "Black Death" which affected most of Europe in the 14th century is generally attributed to plague (technically *Yersinia pestis).* Literature offers numerous examples of such episodes of widespread contagion.

Influenza is a virus that causes respiratory disease in humans, with typical symptoms of fever, cough, and muscle aches, and, rarely, pneumonia and death. Though primarily a human pathogen, influenza viruses also circulate and cause illness in swine, horses, mink, seals, and domestic poultry, and may be carried without apparent illness in these species as well as a number of species of waterfowl.[5] Influenza is highly contagious in humans, spreading through direct contact and aerosol exposure. The virus can also persist for several hours on inanimate objects such as toys or doorknobs. In addition, influenza is infectious before symptoms appear in its victims, which also enhances its spread.[6]

Influenza viruses have a genome composed of eight segments of RNA. In addition to random mutation, flu viruses also undergo change by shuffling or *reassorting* these gene segments among different strains. Flu strains are identified by two important surface antigens (proteins) that are responsible for virulence: hemagglutinin (H) and neuraminidase (N). Fifteen different H antigens and nine different N antigens have been identified in birds and mammals. Not all possible combinations of H and N antigens have been documented, and very few combinations have been shown to cause human illness. The avian flu strain causing great concern at this time is designated as H5N1 for its surface antigens.

New influenza strains typically circle the globe within three to six months of emergence. New strains circulate each year, changing slightly from prior strains (called *genetic drift)* so that healthy adults have partial immunity to new strains. Each year the virus, its genome in constant flux, typically makes healthy people sick, but is generally not deadly. Now and then, often several times in a century, the virus changes enough through reassortment (called *genetic shift)* that there is no partial immunity in the population. This event, an influenza pandemic, results in severe illness and death, even in healthy people. The extent and severity of illness, and the disabling impact on healthy young people, could cause serious disruptions in services and social order.

In this report, unless otherwise noted, the term *pandemic* will be used to refer to pandemic influenza.

Pandemic Phases

According to WHO, the hallmarks of an influenza pandemic are: (1) the emergence of a novel influenza virus strain; (2) the finding that the strain can cause human disease; and (3) sustained person-to-person transmission of the strain. Novel influenza viruses typically acquire these characteristics in phases. Table 1 shows the phases of an influenza pandemic as described by WHO. In the *interpandemic period*, there is no human circulation of novel viruses. During this period, there is annual circulation of common influenza viruses, which cause outbreaks each winter. In the *pandemic alert period,* a new strain is present, with increasing ability for human-to-human spread. During a *pandemic period* there is sustained human-to-human transmission of the new strain. Table 1 also shows the public health goals WHO recommends to slow the development and spread of novel virus strains as much as possible. WHO notes that with respect to the H5N1 avian flu currently circulating, "the level of pandemic alert remains unchanged at phase 3: a virus new to humans is causing infections, but does not spread easily from one person to another."[7]

Influenza Pandemics in the 20th Century[8]

Historical records suggest that influenza pandemics have occurred periodically for at least four centuries. In the 20th century there were three influenza pandemics, and three "pandemic scares."

The **1918 Spanish Flu** (H1N1) pandemic is estimated to have killed between 20 and 100 million people worldwide and at least 500,000 in the United States.[9] Illness and death rates were highest among adults 20-50 years old. HHS notes that "the severity of that virus has not been seen again." Similarities between the 1918 pandemic and the current H5N1 avian flu situation have the global public health community on edge.

Table 1. WHO Pandemic Phases (Revised 2005)

Phase	Description	Overarching public health goals
Interpandemic period		
Phase 1	No new influenza virus strains have been detected in humans. A virus strain that has caused human infection may be present in animals. If so, the risk of human infection is considered to be low.	Strengthen global influenza pandemic preparedness at the global, regional and national levels.
Phase 2	No new influenza virus strains have been detected in humans. However, a circulating animal influenza virus strain poses a substantial risk of human disease.	Minimize the risk of transmission to humans; detect and report such transmission rapidly if it occurs.
Pandemic alert period		
Phase 3	Human infection(s) with a new strain, but no human-to-human spread, or at most rare instances of spread to a close contact.	Ensure rapid characterization of the new virus strain, and early detection, notification and response to additional cases.
Phase 4	Small cluster(s) with limited human-to-human transmission, but spread is highly localized, suggesting that the virus is not well adapted to humans.	Contain the new virus within limited foci or delay spread to gain time to implement preparedness measures, including vaccine development.
Phase 5	Larger cluster(s), but human-to-human spread still localized, suggesting that the virus is becoming increasingly better adapted to humans, but may not yet be fully transmissible (substantial pandemic risk).	Maximize efforts to contain or delay spread, to possibly avert a pandemic, and to gain time to implement pandemic response measures.
Pandemic period		
Phase 6	Pandemic: increased and sustained transmission in the general population	Minimize the impact of the pandemic.

Source: WHO Global Influenza Preparedness Plan, 2005, at [http://www.who.int/csr/disease/influenza/pandemic/en/index.html].

The **1957 Asian Flu** (H2N2) was first identified in Asia in February 1957 and spread to the United States during the summer. Health officials responded quickly and vaccine was available in limited supply by August. This pandemic killed about 69,800 people in the United States.

The **1968 Hong Kong Flu** (H3N2) became widespread in the United States in December of that year. It is estimated that 33,800 people died from this pandemic in the United States, (affecting those over the age of 65 disproportionately), making it the mildest pandemic of the 20th century.

The **1976 Swine Flu** Scare[10] (H1N1) began when a novel virus, identified in New Jersey, was thought to be related to the Spanish flu virus of 1918 and to have pandemic potential. Federal officials mounted a vaccination campaign, and Congress provided liability protection for the manufacturer and federal injury compensation for those harmed by the vaccine. Ultimately, the virus did not spread, but the vaccine was linked with a rare neurological condition that affected more than 500 people and killed 32. The episode damaged confidence in public health officials.

The **1977 Russian Flu** Scare (H1N1) involved a virus strain that had been in circulation prior to 1957. As a result, severe illness was generally limited to those without prior immunity (i.e., children and young adults). The epidemic is not, therefore, considered a true pandemic.

In **1997, H5N1 Avian Flu** emerged in Hong Kong and appeared to have been stamped out by mass culling of poultry. The virus re-emerged in 2003, and global preparedness efforts continue.

In **1999,** an **H9N2 flu** strain was found to have caused human illness in Hong Kong. This strain continues to circulate in birds and remains of concern to public health officials, but has not as yet shown the same lethal potential as the H5N1 strain. In August, 2004, the National Institutes of Health (NIH) awarded a contract to the Chiron corporation to produce up to 40,000 doses of an investigational vaccine against this strain, should it develop the capacity for human-to-human transmission.[11]

Current Situation

H5N1 Avian Influenza

WHO maintains a Web page with a cumulative count of human H5N1 cases.[12] As of November 1, 2005, WHO reported 122 cases, 62 of whom have died, in four countries: Cambodia, Indonesia, Thailand and Vietnam. The WHO describes pandemic influenza and the current situation with H5N1 as follows:[13]

> ... outbreaks ... caused by H5N1 are of particular concern because of their association with severe illness and a high case fatality. Of even greater concern is the uniqueness of the present H5N1 situation in Asia. Never

> before has an avian influenza virus with a documented ability to infect humans caused such widespread outbreaks in birds in so many countries. This unprecedented situation has significantly increased the risk for the emergence of an influenza pandemic.
> ... The risk (of a pandemic) ... remains so long as H5N1 is present in an animal reservoir, thus allowing continuing opportunities for human exposure and infection. ... Most experts agree that control of the present outbreaks in poultry will take several months or even years. ... The recent detection of highly pathogenic avian influenza in wild birds adds another layer of complexity to control.
> ... The world may therefore remain on the verge of a pandemic for some time to come. At the same time, the unpredictability of influenza viruses and the speed with which transmissibility can improve means that the time for preparedness planning is right now. Such a task takes on added urgency because of the prospects opened by recent research: good planning and preparedness might mitigate the enormous consequences of a pandemic, and this opportunity must not be missed.

The H5N1 strain now circulating has been especially virulent in both human and avian hosts. Laboratory studies suggest that the virus prompts an over-reaction of the inflammatory response in humans, causing rapid and severe damage to the lungs.[14] This primary damage cannot be remedied with antibiotics or antiviral drugs. Victims may require mechanical ventilation, and may succumb despite swift and capable care. In 2004, scientists published the results of research in which they sequenced several genes from the 1918 pandemic strains. These genes, when inserted into flu viruses and used to infect mice, were found to have a similar property.[15] Recently, scientists re-created and published the entire genome of the 1918 strain, reinforcing this finding.[16] This property may explain the high lethality of both the 1918 and H5N1 strains in apparently healthy young people.

The H5N1 avian flu may never slip its moorings as a bird pathogen and become a serious human threat. But that possibility is a worst-case scenario for the world's public health experts. Should H5N1 become a pandemic strain, scientists are concerned that it may retain much of its virulence as it changes to a more transmissible form. In the face of such a deadly pathogen, miracles of modern medicine, unavailable in much of the developing world, may not be of much help in developed countries either. Such a scenario would challenge governments around the globe.

Other Flu Strains with Pandemic Potential

While H5N1 is the most worrisome, it is not the only recent flu strain with pandemic potential. Several novel strains of avian influenza associated with human transmission have resulted in pandemic alert status in the past several years. For example, in 2003 an H7N7 strain affecting commercial poultry flocks in the Netherlands resulted in 89 cases of human illness.[17] Most illnesses were mild, but there was one death. In 2004 in the Canadian province of British Columbia, an H7N3 avian influenza strain in commercial poultry was found to have infected at least two people. While both recovered, WHO issued a pandemic alert for the Canadian outbreak.[18]

A government worker who became ill while involved in culling flocks of poultry during an outbreak of H7N2 avian flu in Virginia was later shown to have antibodies to that strain, providing suggestive but not conclusive evidence of infection.[19] This and other cases demonstrate a newer understanding of the potential for direct bird-to-human transmission of avian flu viruses, and the fact that while the H5N1 strain is of special concern, public health officials can not neglect other strains. The Centers for Disease Control and Prevention (CDC) has noted several outbreaks of various strains of avian flu in North American poultry flocks in 2003 and 2004, and publishes guidance and recommendations for the protection of persons potentially exposed during such outbreaks.[20]

Potential Impacts of an Influenza Pandemic

Deaths and Hospitalizations

A WHO influenza expert has said that estimates of the global death toll from a future pandemic are “all over the place.”[21] The WHO estimates that, in the best case, there would be 2 million deaths worldwide from a possible influenza pandemic, and, in the worst case, more than 50 million.[22] In its final pandemic flu plan, HHS estimates that about 209,000 U.S. deaths could result from a moderate pandemic, similar to those in 1957 and 1968, while 1.9 million deaths could result from a severe pandemic like that in 1918.[23] (CDC estimates that on average, about 36,000 die of influenza during an annual flu season.)

Estimates of impacts of a future pandemic are generally based on experience from past pandemics, which varied considerably in their severity. Trust for America’s Health (TFAH), a non-profit public health advocacy group, published a report estimating deaths and hospitalizations in the United States based on mild, moderate and severe pandemic scenarios. The report presents death estimates that range from 180,000 to more than 1 million.[24] The report also contains estimated state-by-state health impacts.

Predicted hospitalization rates provide an idea of the potential burden on the U.S. healthcare system, but they are prone to the same degree of uncertainty. In its final pandemic plan, HHS estimates of hospitalizations range from 865,000 to 9.9 million. TFAH estimates that U.S. hospitalizations would range from almost 800,000 to more than 4.7 million, and cites a statistic from the American Hospital Association that in 2003 there were 965,256 staffed hospital beds in registered hospitals. These projected impacts would occur over a compressed time frame of several weeks or a few months, rather than spread over a full year.

Simple extrapolations of health effects from events in 1918 do not account for advances in medical care that have occurred since then. Antibiotics are now available to treat bacterial pneumonia that often results from influenza infection, and sophisticated respiratory care is now available to treat those with severe pneumonia. Experts caution, though, that the H5N1 avian flu virus can cause severe primary damage to the lungs. If this strain were to launch a pandemic and retain this trait, large numbers of victims may require intensive care and ventilatory support, likely exceeding national capacity to provide this level of care. In any event, such specialized care is not available in most developing countries, and access to it is uneven within the United States.

An influenza pandemic of even limited magnitude has the potential to disrupt the normal workings of the healthcare system in a variety of ways. These may include deferral of elective medical procedures; diversion of patients away from overwhelmed hospital emergency departments and tertiary care facilities; protective quarantines of susceptible populations such as residents of long-term care facilities; and hoarding, theft or black-marketeering of scarce resources such as vaccines or antiviral drugs.

Several additional factors complicate the healthcare burden posed by pandemic flu. First, it is thought that a pandemic would spread across the United States in a compressed timeframe similar to seasonal flu, that is, over a six to eight week period. Second, while it is desirable that affected patients be kept in isolation, domestic isolation capacity is limited. Third, the healthcare workforce is likely to be affected by pandemic flu. Even if they are protected directly by limited vaccines or antiviral drugs, their family members may be affected and require additional care at home. Fourth, supplies of healthcare consumables such as gloves, masks and antibiotics would be stressed by a surge in global demand. Even a mild flu pandemic would likely place a significant and near-simultaneous strain on the nation's healthcare system.

Economic Impacts

There are few estimates of the potential economic impact of a flu pandemic. An analysis published by CDC in 1999, based on the relatively mild 1968 pandemic, estimated the cost of a pandemic in the United States at between $71.3 and $166.5 billion.[25] The study modeled direct healthcare costs, lost productivity for those affected, and lost expected future lifetime earnings for those who died. Loss of life accounted for the majority of economic impact. The model did not include the potential effect of disruptions in commerce. In a recent analysis, the World Bank estimated the overall U.S. economic impacts of a potential pandemic of moderate severity at $100 to $200 billion, and global impacts at around $800 billion, if certain impacts were to last for a full year.[26]

Several economists studied the economic impacts of Severe Acute Respiratory Syndrome (SARS) in 2003. One analysis showed significant short- and long-term decreases in Gross Domestic Product (GDP) in China and Hong Kong, attributing most of the losses to "the behavior of consumers and investors" rather than to actual medical costs.[27] In May 2003, the Conference Board of Canada estimated that the SARS outbreak in Toronto would lower real GDP in Canada by approximately $1.5 billion, or 0.15 percent, in 2003, projecting that the largest effect would be seen in the travel and tourism industries. Consumer behavior and its economic consequences may be affected by official actions and the response of the news media. Some Canadian officials were critical of a WHO advisory warning against travel to Toronto at the height of the outbreak.[28] The World Bank economic analysis of avian flu discusses the likely interplay between government statements and actions, public behavior, and economic effects.

Pandemic Influenza Preparedness and Response

A serious pandemic would trigger the National Response Plan (NRP), developed by the Department of Homeland Security (DHS) as a blueprint for the coordination of federal agencies during an emergency. The NRP, discussed in greater detail in later sections of this report, is an *all-hazards* plan for emergencies ranging from hurricanes to wildfires to terrorist attacks.

Described below are a number of strategies and operational plans to assist countries and U.S. federal, state and local agencies in preparing specifically for a flu pandemic. U.S. plans are intended to reflect the time lines, goals and international capabilities described by the WHO in its pandemic plan. In addition, U.S. federal, state and local plans for this specific threat are intended to be consistent with the all-hazards principles in the NRP.

WHO Global Influenza Preparedness Plan

In order to guide country planning efforts, the WHO released a revised pandemic preparedness plan in early 2005.[29] The plan lays out goals and actions to be taken by WHO, as well as recommended actions for individual nations, at each of the pandemic phases (shown in Table 1). For each phase, actions are grouped into five categories: (1) planning and coordination; (2) situation monitoring and assessment; (3) prevention and containment; (4) health system response; and (5) communications. In addition, recommended actions for individual nations are grouped according to whether the country is affected or not at a particular phase. For Phase 6 (Pandemic Phase), when it is assumed that all countries will inevitably be affected, there are recommended immediate actions for all countries, and specific actions for those affected, those not yet affected, and those for which the pandemic has subsided, noting that subsequent pandemic waves may follow the first one.

The WHO pandemic plan contains an annex of recommendations to nations for "nonpharmaceutical public health interventions," actions such as isolation, quarantine and travel restrictions. The annex stresses the use of voluntary rather than compulsory measures, noting the lack of demonstrated utility of certain practices, or that enforcement is considered impractical for others. The annex also notes that certain practices used to control SARS, such as temperature screening at airports, are not necessarily recommended for control of pandemic influenza, depending on pandemic phase. (Because influenza virus is more transmissible than SARS, some SARS control measures are not considered effective for flu.) The plan and annex also stress avoiding stigmatization of persons affected by pandemic influenza or its control measures.

HHS Draft Pandemic Plan

In August 2004, HHS released a draft pandemic influenza preparedness and response plan.[30] The draft plan articulated steps to be taken by HHS agencies and offices, and by state and local public health authorities, in preparing for and responding to a pandemic. Specific activities discussed included surveillance, vaccine development and use, antiviral drug use, and communications. The draft plan was criticized by some as being vague, and for delegating certain critical activities — such as designating priority groups for rationing of vaccine and antiviral drugs — to states.[31]

National Strategy for Pandemic Influenza

On November 1, 2005, the administration released a "National Strategy for Pandemic Influenza," on a central website containing interagency pandemic preparedness and response information.[32] The strategy lays out three goals: (1) stopping, slowing or otherwise limiting the spread of a pandemic to the United States; (2) limiting the domestic spread of a pandemic, and mitigating disease, suffering and death; and (3) sustaining infrastructure and mitigating impact to the economy and the functioning of society. In order to meet those goals, the strategy lays out three "pillars" of implementation activities:

- Preparedness and Communication: Activities that should be undertaken before a pandemic to ensure preparedness, and the communication of roles and responsibilities to all levels of government, segments of society and individuals.
- Surveillance and Detection: Domestic and international systems that provide continuous "situational awareness," to ensure the earliest warning possible to protect the population.
- Response and Containment: Actions to limit the spread of the outbreak and to mitigate the health, social and economic impacts of a pandemic.

Finally, roles and responsibilities are laid out for the federal government, state and local governments, the private sector, individuals and families, and international partners.

In announcing the strategic plan, President Bush sent a budget request to Congress seeking $7.1 billion in emergency spending for the departments of

HHS, Agriculture, Defense, Homeland Security, Interior, State and Veterans Affairs.[33] The proposed funding would: (1) support enhanced domestic and international planning and surveillance activities ($259 million requested); (2) purchase stockpiles of vaccines and antiviral drugs, and accelerate the development of new vaccine technologies ($6.242 billion requested); and (3) aid in federal, state and local preparedness efforts ($644 million requested.)

HHS Final Pandemic Plan

HHS released its final pandemic influenza plan on November 2, 2005.[34] The final plan builds on elements in the draft plan, and has three parts: (1) a Strategic Plan, which outlines key planning assumptions and HHS agency roles; (2) a Public Health Guidance for State and Local Partners, which lays out activities on such matters as surveillance, laboratory testing, and quarantine at the borders; and (3) a part currently under development, to consist of detailed operational plans for HHS agencies involved in pandemic response. According to the plan, the HHS Secretary would direct, and the Assistant Secretary for Public Health Emergency Preparedness would coordinate, all HHS pandemic response activities.

The final plan will be critiqued over time. Some concerns with the draft plan have been addressed, such as the designation of priority groups to receive limited vaccine and antiviral drugs.[35] Other elements of the final plan received immediate criticism. For example, the section on healthcare planning focuses on individual healthcare facilities and refers to plans for surge capacity. Some experts have commented that there is little surge capacity in the healthcare sector under normal circumstances, and that officials might have to resort to the use of alternate facilities (e.g., convention centers) to care for large numbers of flu patients. The HHS final plan does not address that contingency.

Department of Defense Planning and Activities

Shortly after the release of the HHS draft pandemic plan in August 2004, the Assistant Secretary of Defense for Health Affairs released the Department of Defense (DOD) "Pandemic Influenza Preparation and Response Planning Guidance."[36] The DOD guidance follows many of the assumptions used in the civilian plan, modifying them to protect a highly mobile military force during wartime. Frequent mention is made of the extremely high mortality suffered by U.S. troops during World War I as a result of the 1918 pandemic. The guidance notes that 43,000 uniformed soldiers, more than one third of all U.S. military casualties in the war, died of pandemic influenza, most of them during one 10-week period in 1918.

The DOD guidance notes that the military will use the same vaccine formulation as that developed for civilian use, though DOD will be responsible for securing its own supplies of vaccine and antiviral drugs. Priority for countermeasures in limited supply would be given to forward-deployed troops. The guidance does not set out strict tiers of priority recipients (nor had the HHS draft plan). The guidance discusses the limited utility of individual control measures such as isolation and quarantine, and suggests that larger-scale adjustments (such as extending the tour of ships at sea) could slow disease transmission. The guidance also mentions the consideration of coalition forces from other nations, and the possibility that countermeasures such as vaccine and antiviral drugs may be provided to them under certain conditions.

On November 7, 2005, DOD's Deployment Health Support Directorate announced a new website to provide service members with information on avian and pandemic influenza.[37] The Department has not publicly released a revised or final version of its 2004 pandemic flu guidance.

DOD maintains the Global Emerging Infectious Diseases Surveillance program (GEIS), which has long been a source of year-round global influenza surveillance data.[38] The guidance states that DOD will provide information gleaned from this system, as well as its global laboratory network, to WHO and CDC officials tracking pre-pandemic and pandemic flu virus activity.

Department of Veterans Affairs Planning and Activities

The Department of Veterans Affairs (VA) notes that it is involved in coordinated pandemic influenza planning, though limited information is publicly available.[39] Pandemic planning activities are to be expansions of the department's seasonal flu control activities, which include vaccination programs and surveillance. To date, the VA has stockpiled 550,000 treatment courses of the antiviral drug, Tamiflu.

State Pandemic Preparedness Plans

All states were required to have submitted plans for pandemic flu preparedness to HHS (through CDC) by July 2005, as a condition of receipt of public health preparedness funding for FY2005.[40] CDC reports that it has received plans from all states.[41] As of October 2005, 32 states had posted draft or final plans on a public website.[42] Of these, 15 state plans were dated within 2005, and the remainder earlier. Since states were required to submit their plans before a final federal plan was available, some states may subsequently update their plans to reflect new planning information.

Guidance provided by CDC directed states to incorporate the following elements in their pandemic influenza preparedness plans:

- Assemble an executive planning committee;
- Identify and meet with partners and stakeholders;
- Establish command, control and management procedures;
- Establish procedures for essential functions: surveillance and laboratory testing; delivery of vaccines and antiviral drugs; emergency health and medical response; maintenance of essential services; and communications.[43]

The Association of State and Territorial Health Officials (ASTHO) also produced a guidance document to assist its members in developing plans.[44] In addition to activities described in the CDC guidance, the ASTHO document contains a checklist of additional tasks in pandemic planning, including:

- A review of state policies and authorities regarding public health and medical issues such as: quarantine; mandatory vaccination; the closure of schools and businesses; volunteer licensure, liability and compensation; and the use of temporary medical facilities.
- A review of state authorities and individuals responsible for issues outside the public health and medical sphere, such as: establishing incident command; coordinating activities across state agencies, and with health agencies in adjacent states; and use of law enforcement and National Guard support.

Issues in Pandemic Influenza Planning

Could an Influenza Pandemic be Stopped?

Public health experts note that vaccine, the primary measure for influenza prevention, will be available in very limited supply at the start of any pandemic, and is unlikely ever to be available to everyone. Antiviral drugs are also likely to be available in a limited supply. For both, there is limited global surge capacity for production during a pandemic. Conventional wisdom once held that there was an inevitability to the global wave of disease that a pandemic would bring, but lately this notion has been challenged. WHO and many national experts believe that scientific advances in studying and detecting flu viruses may make it possible to detect the spread of the virus early and rein in localized clusters of infection. While not suggesting that a pandemic could necessarily be averted, they posit that if progression were slowed enough, a vaccine could be available by the time worldwide infection ensued. While there still might not be enough vaccine for everyone, if countries had at least enough for essential personnel, it would soften the impact somewhat.

Realizing this hope rests on two conditions: first, exceptional "pandemic intelligence" in countries at the epicenter of a developing pandemic; and second, priority use of control measures in these epicenter countries. In hopes of having the best possible information in real time, WHO, CDC, and health officials from many other nations are building epidemiology and lab capacity in Southeast Asian countries affected by H5N1 avian flu, when those countries have requested assistance. This aid is layered onto an uneven patchwork of existing capacities. In supplemental appropriations for FY2005 (P.L. 109-13), Congress provided $15 million (through the foreign assistance account at the State Department) to supplement CDC's existing activities to expand epidemiology and laboratory capacity in that region.

The second requirement for successful pre-pandemic containment, namely priority use of control measures in affected countries, is politically difficult. It would require that countries contribute vaccine and antiviral drugs to a global stockpile to be used in epicenter countries to slow a pandemic. Costs notwithstanding, given that countries would face severe shortages of these precious assets if a pandemic reaches them, would they share their national stockpiles with other countries? Many U.S. analysts believe that doing so is not merely altruistic. They argue that providing antiviral drugs to an affected country in the early going would save American lives in the long run. While plausible, this thesis is untested, and

WHO has had limited success to date in getting nations to commit assets to the global stockpile.

Who's in Charge?

The National Response Plan (NRP) published by DHS, is a blueprint for the coordinated efforts of federal agencies during disasters.[45] In the event of a significant influenza pandemic, the NRP may be activated to coordinate federal agency activities. Responsibilities for specified activities (e.g., transportation, energy, and public works) are set out in 15 *Emergency Support Functions* (ESF). When asked who would be in the lead for the federal response during a pandemic, Dr. Jeffrey Runge, Chief Medical Officer for DHS, replied:

> When critical infrastructures are threatened, the secretary of DHS is responsible for the preservation of critical infrastructures. HHS will continue to have the lead in prevention, containment and treatment of avian flu. But if the government surges, and if the ESFs (Emergency Support Functions) stand up and so forth, the secretary of DHS will be responsible for each of those emergency support functions discharging their duty. One of the duties of HHS is containment, prevention and treatment of avian flu.[46]

When the NRP is activated, the Secretary of Homeland Security serves as the overall lead for a coordinated federal response, while the Secretary of HHS serves as the lead for ESF#8, Public Health and Medical Services.[47] While public health and medical activities may comprise the bulk of the federal response to a pandemic, other ESF authorities may be involved to sustain infrastructure affected by absenteeism or supply chain disruptions, requiring the coordination of other federal departments.

Overarching federal leadership in DHS may be called upon to address problems such as the prioritization of federal non-medical resources, if these resources were exhausted by demands from many states simultaneously. State disaster planning commonly relies on state-to-state mutual aid, in addition to federal assistance.[48] In a severe pandemic, assistance from other states may be limited, and federal assistance may be thinly stretched.

The NRP is intended to identify federal roles and leadership for a *response* to an emergency, and resolve coordination difficulties. Experience gained from the implementation of the NRP after Hurricane Katrina indicates that there may be a gap in leadership for *preparedness*.

WHO urges that countries plan for a pandemic as a multi-sector threat, not merely a health challenge. Planning in HHS and state health agencies is ongoing, but some assert that a clear point of leadership is needed at the federal level to engage state, local and municipal officials in multi-sector planning. The National Strategy notes that lead departments have been identified for the medical response (HHS), veterinary response (Department of Agriculture), international activities (Department of State) and overall domestic incident management (DHS). Each of these departments would serve as the federal liaison to assist its respective sectors in planning. In addition, DHS is responsible for coordinating the preparedness of privately owned critical infrastructures such as banking or telecommunications.

However, federal relationships that support state and local jurisdictions traditionally operate sector-by-sector (e.g., HHS with health services, and the Department of Transportation with transit agencies). At this time, a mayor would have difficulty identifying one point of contact concerning the spectrum of planning activities that would be needed to keep water running, lights on, food stocked, and gasoline flowing during a serious flu pandemic. Further, while pandemic influenza scenarios have been used to exercise specific elements of response, such as distribution of stockpiled medications, there has been no large-scale exercise to study a coordinated, multi-sector response to this potential nationwide threat.[49]

Emergency Declarations and Federal Assistance

In the United States, public health authority rests principally with the states as an exercise of their *police powers*.[50] States play a leading role in preparing for and responding to public health threats, with HHS (primarily CDC) providing support through funding, training, technical assistance, advanced laboratory support, data analysis and other activities. The Public Health Service Act grants the Secretary of HHS the authority to declare a situation a public health emergency, which triggers an expansion of certain federal authorities.[51] Though states already have considerable power in responding to public health events, most can also declare public health emergencies and expand their powers further. In an influenza pandemic, response measures such as quarantine or prohibitions against administration of vaccine to non-priority individuals would likely be carried out, at least initially, by state rather than federal authorities.[52]

An influenza pandemic may disrupt services beyond the health sector. A multi-sector federal response to a pandemic could be directed by provisions in the NRP. Both the HHS pandemic plan and the DOD pandemic guidance are written with the premise that the NRP would be triggered by a severe influenza pandemic, thereby guiding a coordinated federal response to problems within the health sector and other sectors that may be affected, through routine (non-emergency) federal assistance mechanisms. The Biological Incident Annex in the NRP notes that "Actions described in this annex take place with or without a Presidential Stafford Act declaration or a public health emergency declaration by the Secretary of (HHS)."[53] While the annex addresses intentional bioterrorism events, it also addresses naturally occurring biological threats such as pandemic influenza.

States may require additional federal assistance to maintain essential services during an influenza pandemic. Typically, such assistance is triggered by Presidential emergency or disaster declarations under the Stafford Act.[54] Disaster assistance authorized by the Stafford Act includes the provision of emergency funds and supplies to stricken households as well as aid in clearing and rebuilding damaged infrastructure. While a virus would not cause such damage directly, certain sectors may nonetheless be affected as a result of widespread absenteeism or supply chain disruptions. For example, water treatment facilities may be damaged, or may have to be shut down, if they are not adequately maintained, or if replacement parts are unavailable. Sectors which depend heavily on continuous computer support (e.g., banking) may be disrupted by absenteeism.

Some may question whether the Stafford Act is an appropriate legislative base for action in the event of a flu pandemic. In a recent terrorism preparedness exercise, TOPOFF III, concerns were raised that because the Stafford Act explicitly defines a "major disaster" as a *natural* catastrophe, states facing a terrorism incident would not be eligible for the full range of federal disaster assistance authorized by the act.[55] Such concerns may be met, however, with the recognition that the definition of the term "emergency" in the statute provides greater discretion to the President in issuing an emergency declaration. However, pursuant to the Stafford Act, considerably less financial assistance may be provided under an emergency declaration, compared to that authorized under a major disaster declaration.

An influenza pandemic may pose a challenge in national disaster response that is without recent precedent. A pandemic could affect all or almost all areas of the United States with multi-sector impacts within a six to eight week period, involving the entire country nearly at once. A severe pandemic could cause "extraordinary levels of mass casualties" and substantial disruptions in services, and thereby meet the definition of a *Catastrophic Incident* according to the NRP.[56] Questions might be raised about the adequacy of the Catastrophic Incident Annex in the NRP. The Annex was not activated during the response to Hurricane Katrina.[57] DHS officials have said that the Annex and related planning documents are not yet complete.[58]

Limited Surveillance and Detection Capability

The CDC coordinates domestic surveillance for seasonal flu. Monitoring for pandemic flu is integrated into these existing systems. Key challenges in the rapid detection of novel flu viruses are the vagueness of flu symptoms, which can be seen with many other diseases, and the difficulty in distinguishing specific strains of interest from the background of other flu strains commonly in circulation.

The routine CDC system for domestic flu surveillance has seven reporting components: (1) more than 120 laboratories; (2) more than 1,000 sentinel healthcare providers; (3) death records from 122 cities; (4) reports from health departments in the states, territories, New York City and the District of Columbia; (5) influenza-associated deaths in children; (6) Emerging Infections Program sites in 10 states; and (7) laboratory-confirmed hospitalizations of young children in three sentinel counties.[59] Reporting to these systems by state and local health departments and healthcare providers is voluntary. Information is gathered and analyzed weekly during the winter flu season. The final HHS pandemic plan proposes that BioSense, a new system to gather, in real time, information such as emergency department admissions, be incorporated along with other flu detection systems.

Through the Health Alert Network, CDC has issued recommendations to public health and medical professionals, addressing domestic surveillance and laboratory investigation of possible cases of avian or pandemic influenza.[60] CDC recommends that health professionals use screening tests for influenza on individuals who have a history of recent travel to an affected region and exhibit symptoms of severe respiratory disease. Specimens that test positive on screening for influenza should be followed up with samples sent to CDC to determine which flu strain is involved. CDC is working with states to develop state-based lab capability for testing flu viruses for the H5 antigen, but this capability is not yet in place.[61]

Isolation and Quarantine

Isolation and quarantine have been used for hundreds of years to prevent the spread of communicable diseases. Both methods restrict the movement of those affected, but they differ depending on whether an individual has been exposed to a disease (*quarantine*), or is actually infected (*isolation*). Persons in isolation may be significantly ill, so isolation often occurs in a healthcare setting. Persons under quarantine are, by definition, not ill from the disease in question, though they may have other health conditions that complicate the quarantine process.

In the United States, quarantine authority is generally based in state rather than federal law.[62] The federal government has the responsibility to prevent the introduction, transmission, and spread of communicable diseases from foreign countries, and the authority to impose quarantine on incoming travelers suspected to be infected with or exposed to certain diseases on a list of quarantinable communicable diseases. Diseases are listed by an executive order of the President, in consultation with the Secretary of HHS. On April 1, 2005, President Bush added to the list "influenza caused by novel or re-emergent influenza viruses that are causing, or have the potential to cause, a pandemic."[63] Federal quarantine is carried out by CDC's Division of Global Migration and Quarantine, which operates quarantine stations at major ports, and also works closely with states to carry out quarantine activities.[64] CDC has noted that having pandemic influenza on the list assures the agency of this option for disease control, should it be felt to be worthwhile.

On October 4, 2005, in response to a question at a press conference, President Bush suggested the use of the military to enforce quarantines during a flu pandemic.[65] The comment prompted responses on two issues: the role of the military in domestic disasters, and the role of quarantine in controlling pandemic flu.

Following the terror attacks of 2001, in October of 2002, DOD activated a new combatant command, Northern Command or NORTHCOM, to, among other functions, provide military assistance to civil authorities in response to terrorist attacks.[66] The NRP also articulates this role for the military in response to terrorist attacks, major disasters, and other emergencies.[67] There has, however, long been a prohibition against the use of federal military personnel for domestic law enforcement, except in extraordinary circumstances.[68] There are no instances in the 20th century in which federal troops were used to enforce a domestic quarantine for any disease, though there are earlier examples.[69] On October 13, 2005,

Assistant Secretary of Defense for Homeland Defense Paul McHale commented that the threshold for use of troops during a domestic disaster would be high, but that "... an outbreak of avian flu could be so severe that active-duty forces might need to help the National Guard enforce quarantines," and that " ... Congress and federal agencies must establish clear guidelines on what would trigger a broad U.S. military response to restore law and order."[70]

While isolation and quarantine were crucial in the worldwide response to SARS, these methods are less likely to be successful in controlling influenza. Influenza is more highly contagious than SARS, has a shorter incubation period, and is often contagious in the absence of symptoms or before symptoms appear, making it difficult to identify persons who should be quarantined.[71] Public health officials have suggested the use of quarantines in certain circumstances (e.g., incoming passenger flights) to delay the emergence of pandemic influenza in an area, but have generally steered away from suggesting the more traditional use of quarantine of individuals as a containment measure for pandemic flu, recommending instead the use of voluntary, population-based approaches (e.g., cancelling sporting events).[72]

Rationing Scarce Resources

The WHO recommends that countries identify priority groups for vaccination and antiviral drugs (as these measures become available) and that countries make these decisions before a pandemic occurs. The National Vaccine Advisory Committee (NVAC, which reports to the director of the National Vaccine Program in HHS) and the Advisory Committee on Immunization Practices (ACIP, which reports to the HHS Secretary and CDC) met in joint session in July 2005 to report to HHS Secretary Leavitt their recommendations for prioritizing vaccine and antiviral drugs for the U.S. civilian population during a pandemic.[73] The two committees concurred on each group's unanimous recommendations for prioritizing pandemic flu vaccine. Their recommendations were incorporated into the HHS final pandemic plan, and are displayed in Table 2.

Healthcare workers with direct patient contact and those involved in making the vaccine were given top priority by the committees. Next were those at highest risk of serious complications from flu. During seasonal flu, and during the 1957 and 1968 pandemics, those at highest risk were the very old, the very young, and individuals with certain serious chronic diseases.

The committees noted that during a pandemic other groups may be shown to be at higher risk, and that tiers could be redefined according to the specific epidemiologic findings. For example, during the 1918 pandemic, healthy young people were found to be at increased risk of death when they became infected. According to the committees' estimates, more than 60% of the U.S. population would not fall into any of the designated priority groups.

Table 2. NVAC and ACIP Recommendations for Pandemic Vaccine Priority Groups (persons in thousands)

Group and Tier	Group total	Cumulative total
1A. Healthcare workers with direct patient contact	9,000	9,000
Vaccine and antivirals manufacturing personnel	40	9,040
1B. Highest risk of serious flu complications	25,840	34,880
1C. Pregnant women, immunocompromised individuals, and household contacts of infants	10,700	45,580
1D. Key government leaders and responders	151	45,731
2A. Rest of high risk individuals	59,100	104,831
2B. Most critical infrastructure and public health emergency responders	8,500	113,331
3. Other key government health decision makers, mortuary services personnel	500	113,831
4. Healthy 2-64 yr. olds not in other groups	179,260	293,091

While the proposed scheme emphasizes the protection of those who are most vulnerable to severe complications from flu, it does not necessarily reflect the goal of saving the most lives. To achieve the latter when resources are scarce, treatment would be given to those most likely to have better outcomes as a result. Conversely, treatment could be withheld from those who are unlikely to benefit, so that others may. These are ethically complex decisions with which the civilian medical community has little experience. Also, in this case, science does not provide ready answers.

In 2005, both the peer-reviewed medical literature and the popular press have carried numerous reports about the possibility of decreasing societal flu transmission by vaccinating children, and of possibly limited effectiveness of flu vaccine in the frail or institutionalized elderly. The science leaves policymakers uncertain on both counts. Available studies are limited and conflicting, often with non-comparable designs, and they are observational rather than controlled. (Controlled studies of such questions could violate ethical standards and guidelines for the protection of study subjects.)

Lacking better evidence to guide decisions, some are left with a sense of unease as they try to envision which groups should receive flu vaccine during a pandemic.[74]

Influenza Vaccine Supply and Use

Limited Vaccine Production Capacity

Vaccination is considered the best preventive measure for influenza. Flu vaccine is currently produced in chicken eggs in a time-consuming process with a six-month lead time.[75] Since a vaccine could not be mass produced against a pandemic flu strain until that strain emerged, planning assumes that flu vaccine will not be available for initial global pandemic control.[76] Nonetheless, health officials are working to increase the speed of flu vaccine production, to increase global flu vaccine production capacity, and to ready candidate vaccines for H5N1 and H9N2 avian flu, in the event that either of these were to become a pandemic strain.

Currently, there is worldwide capacity to produce at most 300 million doses of *trivalent* flu vaccine, the annual vaccine that contains three different strains of influenza.[77] Only one (sanofi Pasteur[78]) of nine manufacturers of injectable flu vaccine is located in the United States. Capacity for this producer is expected to be approximately 60 million trivalent doses for 2005-2006.

Though production capacity can, in theory, be tripled by converting to single-strain production for a pandemic vaccine, two doses (vs. the single dose given each year) may be required to afford protection, because there is no prior immunity to be "boosted." Furthermore, in initial trials of an H5N1 prototype vaccine, immunity was produced only by very high doses of viral antigen, which means that more capacity would be needed to make a given number of doses.

The President's supplemental budget request for pandemic flu says, "The centerpiece of the (HHS) proposal is to increase vaccine manufacturing capacity to allow for the production of pandemic influenza vaccine for the entire nation within a six-month period... ."[79] The request mentions the possible use of the funds for renovation and construction, and for research, but lacks additional detail regarding how federal funds might be used to build private capacity for this crucial but rarely needed intervention. On November 2, 2005, HHS Secretary Leavitt testified that HHS would pursue a multi-pronged strategy to increase domestic production capacity and stockpile expansion, with goals to be achieved in phases between 2008 and

2013. The stated goals include (1) licensing additional domestic manufacturers of injectable flu vaccine; (2) transitioning from egg-based to cell-based production; and (3) research in new vaccine technologies.[80]

Leavitt stated that HHS would support research on the use of *adjuvants* (i.e., vaccine additives that boost immunity), lowering the needed dose of virus, and thereby stretching available capacity. One expert has commented that if the United States had prioritized the use of adjuvants sooner, it could be farther along in establishing not only adequate domestic capacity for pandemic vaccine production, but also added capacity to assist other nations that lack capacity of their own.[81] He proposed that under optimal conditions, if all the world's vaccine companies were to use a certain adjuvant to produce pandemic flu vaccines, that within six months' time there could be enough vaccine for 3.6 billion people, about half the world's population.

The use of adjuvants in flu vaccine would add additional scientific, technical and regulatory obstacles, especially new safety concerns. For this reason, the United States has developed prototype H5N1 vaccines using methods similar to those used for seasonal vaccine production, an approach that would optimize the chances for success in the near-term, in the event that a pandemic were imminent.

Regulatory Issues

From a regulatory standpoint, the Food and Drug Administration (FDA) considers that a pandemic flu vaccine produced using currently-approved processes would merely represent a strain change (as with seasonal flu vaccine), not a new product.[82] This would allow for a streamlined approval process in which a licensed manufacturer would submit additional information as a supplement to its current product license. The agency considers that virus derived by reverse genetics or grown using cell culture methods does not pose additional regulatory obstacles.[83] Prototype human vaccines ideally should undergo clinical trials to establish efficacy, dosage and scheduling protocols. The FDA recommends that these trials be carried out before any pandemic occurs, to the extent possible.

The National Institutes of Health (NIH) has awarded contracts to Aventis Pasteur (now sanofi pasteur) to develop prototype human vaccines against H5N1 flu, and to Chiron Corporation to develop vaccines against H5N1 as well as H9N2 flu.[84] Clinical trials of these vaccines are ongoing, under NIH supervision.

The HHS final plan notes that if a pandemic were to spread swiftly, pandemic vaccine may be pressed into service before standard safety and efficacy tests could be completed. Such unlicensed vaccine could be used under FDA's Investigational New Drug (IND) provisions. These include strict inventory control, record keeping, and informed consent requirements, which would pose an additional challenge for public health officials during a vaccination campaign.

Congress provided an additional mechanism, permitting the use of unapproved drugs and vaccines in an emergency, in the Project BioShield Act of 2004 (P.L. 108-276). This *Emergency Use Authorization* (EUA) permits the use of unapproved products during a declared public health emergency when alternatives are not available.[85] In early 2005, when FDA issued an EUA for an anthrax vaccine for the military, the agency noted that the statute is self-executing, and that implementing regulations were not required.[86]

Liability and Compensation

Certain vaccines are covered under the National Vaccine Injury Compensation Program (VICP). Under VICP, an excise tax applied to vaccine sales pays for a public compensation fund. Congress enacted the program in 1986 as a no-fault alternative to the tort system for resolving personal injury claims resulting from adverse reactions to recommended childhood vaccines. Individuals of any age alleging injury from any covered vaccine must seek compensation through the program first, though they may decline a proposed award and then seek a remedy in court.[87] Congress added *trivalent* flu vaccine (the annual vaccine that contains three strains) to the VICP list in the American Jobs Creation Act of 2004 (P.L.108-357). Since the law explicitly covered trivalent vaccine, *monovalent* (or single-strain) pandemic vaccines would not be covered under VICP. Mechanisms to indemnify manufacturers and officials involved in a pandemic flu vaccine campaign, and to compensate those who may be injured by a monovalent pandemic vaccine, do not exist at this time.

Important lessons from the smallpox vaccination program in 2003 and the swine flu scare in 1976 inform policy discussions about liability and compensation today.

During implementation of the smallpox vaccination program, Congress grappled with the task of waiving liability in order to protect the manufacturer, public officials, health providers and others who would make, recommend and deliver the product, while assuring that those who suffered adverse events resulting from the vaccine could be appropriately compensated.[88] The smallpox vaccine used for the 2003 campaign carries an unusually high risk of adverse events, and most scientists do not believe that a pandemic flu vaccine would carry a comparable risk.

Nonetheless, public health officials recall the outcome of the swine flu campaign in 1976, an event that is often called a debacle.[89] In January 1976, a novel influenza strain ("swine flu") emerged in New Jersey. In March, the Ford Administration announced a campaign to vaccinate the U.S. population by December. On August 18, Congress passed P.L. 94-380, the National Swine Flu Immunization Program of 1976. Among other provisions, the law shielded manufacturers, distributors, and public or private organizations that would administer the vaccine from claims of injury or death that might result, and established that all such claims would be asserted directly against the United States. More than 40 million civilians were vaccinated against swine flu between October 1 and December 16. The campaign was suspended at that time due to several findings of a severe neurological condition, causing paralysis and sometimes death, suspected to have been caused by the vaccine. Meanwhile, a flu pandemic never emerged. The worrisome virus from New Jersey never led to a global pandemic, or even to localized outbreaks. The federal government ultimately paid out $93 million to individuals injured by the vaccine.[90]

Analysts have commented that delays in indemnifying manufacturers threatened the availability of swine flu vaccine in 1976, while delays in providing for injury compensation compromised voluntary participation in the smallpox vaccine campaign in 2003. A successful emergency vaccination campaign may depend on resolving both policy concerns expediently. Several bills have been introduced thus far in the 109th Congress to address liability and/or compensation related to the use of a vaccine developed to prevent pandemic influenza. One measure, the Biodefense and Pandemic Vaccine and Drug Development Act of 2005 (S. 1873), was reported by the Senate Committee on Health, Education, Labor, and Pensions. Others, such as S. 1880 and companion bills S. 1437 and H.R. 3970, have not been acted upon. On November 1, 2005, HHS Secretary Leavitt transmitted to Congress a draft bill that would provide limited immunity to persons involved in the manufacture and administration of a pandemic vaccine. The draft bill does not contain provisions for compensation of persons who may be injured by the product.[91]

Intellectual Property Issues

To produce a vaccine against H5N1 or another pandemic flu strain, scientists start with a virus in circulation, and modify it for mass production. Flu virus for vaccine is grown in fertilized chicken eggs. Avian flu strains must first be weakened, or *attenuated*, or they would kill the chicken embryos. Typically, flu viruses are attenuated using a cumbersome trial-and-error gene swapping process. In developing prototype H5N1 vaccines, the virus was attenuated using a process called *reverse genetics* (RG). RG is a more efficient and reliable means of genetic modification, which removes unwanted genes and substitutes others.

RG is a patented invention. One of the patent holders has waived compensation for production of prototype pandemic flu vaccines and clinical trials. Compensation would have to be paid once a pandemic flu vaccine were to enter commercial production. In the United States, the federal government may use patented processes without consent, as long as the patent holder is appropriately compensated.[92] The situation is more complicated in other countries with vaccine plants (mainly in Europe), and would require that certain agreements among RG patent holders and governments be ironed out before mass production could begin.[93]

Use of RG speeds the process of strain selection, and its patent is not felt to be a substantial obstacle to the development of pandemic flu vaccine in the United States. RG could simplify the production of flu vaccine for seasonal use, too, but there the patent may be an obstacle. Annual flu vaccine is an inexpensive product with a small profit margin. Its limited market attractiveness is cited as one reason for the pharmaceutical industry's limited interest in making it. Some are concerned that the market for annual flu vaccine would not bear the added cost of royalties, and that as a result, improved technologies are not incorporated.[94] Since pandemic vaccine would be made on the existing seasonal flu vaccine infrastructure, this potential obstacle to enhanced seasonal capacity may hamper pandemic preparedness. A similar problem may exist with respect to upgrading the system to use cell culture growth methods instead of eggs.

Antiviral Drug Supply and Use

Since pandemic flu vaccine would be unavailable in the early stages of a pandemic, governments and private parties have been interested in drugs that could treat or prevent serious illness from flu. Because influenza is a virus, antibiotics, which treat bacterial infections, are not effective in treating the direct effects of flu. Two types of antiviral drugs have been developed to treat flu: *adamantanes* and *neuraminidase inhibitors* (NIs).[95] Though both types are used to treat serious infections of seasonal influenza, the H5N1 flu strain has been shown to be resistant to adamantanes. Hence, planning efforts for a possible H5N1 pandemic have focused on NIs. Two NIs are available, and both are licensed by the FDA: oseltamivir (Tamiflu®) and zanamivir (Relenza®). The drugs can be used either for treatment when someone is severely ill with flu, or for prevention in those at risk of severe illness. When used for prevention (also called *prophylaxis*), the drugs must be given for weeks (rather than the five-day treatment regime), as long the flu virus is in circulation. This has implications for stockpiling and for the potential development of viral resistance to the drugs.

In June 2005, it was reported that farmers in China were using the flu antiviral drug amantadine (an adamantane) to treat poultry flocks to prevent avian flu, and that this may have caused the H5N1 strain to become resistant to the drug.[96] Health officials in China and elsewhere denounced the practice. Tamiflu, the more widely available of the two NIs, is thought to be effective against H5N1 flu, but clinical data are limited. As yet, only one case of Tamiflu resistance has been documented in a human H5N1 patient. Scientists caution, though, that resistance could become a greater problem if the drug were pressed into service during an influenza pandemic, especially if it were used for prolonged periods for prophylaxis.[97] Tamiflu resistance has been documented in strains of seasonal influenza that circle the globe each year.

WHO has recommended that countries create stockpiles of NIs to prepare for a pandemic. Tamiflu, which is patent protected until 2016, holds the bulk of the global market share for NIs and has been stockpiled by several nations. The drug company Hoffman-La Roche Inc. ("Roche") is the sole maker of Tamiflu, which it produces in a single plant in Switzerland. The company president has testified that the drug takes about 8 to 12 months to produce and has a few production bottlenecks, including a unique natural starter chemical available only in China, and a potentially explosive step that must be carried out in specialized and costly facilities.[98] He also testified that Roche produced 1.7 million courses of treatment for the 2004-2005 flu season and was working to increase capacity by simplifying production methods, expanding its Swiss facility, and building a second facility in the United States.

Government and private purchases have increased to the point that global production capacity for Tamiflu has been exceeded, and orders are now backlogged. Under pressure to allow other companies to make the drug, Roche had previously asserted that because production was so complicated, the company had not been approached by other interested producers. This has recently changed. The company now reports that it has had many such inquiries, and that it has granted some licenses to allow other manufacturers to make the drug.[99] In addition, the company announced on October 27, 2005, that it would suspend shipments of Tamiflu to non-government U.S. purchasers, to prevent hoarding of the drug by individuals.[100]

Several countries have stockpiled enough Tamiflu to treat one-fifth or more of their populations. The United States has stockpiled 4.3 million treatment courses (enough for about 1.5 percent of the population), with some additional amounts pending delivery.[101] The U.S. stockpile of antiviral drugs is maintained in the Strategic National Stockpile (SNS) of drugs, vaccines, antidotes, medical supplies and other measures which may be needed in a public health emergency. The SNS is managed by CDC.

The HHS final pandemic plan proposes that HHS will stockpile enough antiviral drugs to treat 25% of the U.S. population.[102] Per HHS Secretary Leavitt, emergency supplemental funds requested by the President would be used to meet, by the summer of 2007, "the national goal of having available 81 million courses of antivirals, which would be sufficient to treat 25 percent of the U.S. population (75 million courses) and a reserve supply (6 million courses) that could be used to contain an initial U.S. outbreak."[103] Leavitt said that states were expected to procure 31 million of these courses, for which HHS would reimburse 25 percent of the cost. He stressed the importance of this aspect of state involvement in pandemic preparedness. Some public health officials and Members of Congress protested about the proposed 75 percent state matching requirement, saying that it added an extra burden on top of a proposed $130 million cut in state public health preparedness grants for FY2006.[104]

Priority groups for antiviral drugs are laid out in the HHS final pandemic plan, beginning with treatment for those who are admitted to hospitals with severe illness from flu. Priority categories are otherwise fairly similar to those for vaccine (See Table 2.) encompassing certain groups of high risk individuals as well as healthcare workers and other responders.

Public health officials have cautioned against an over-reliance on antiviral drugs in planning, in part because there will be limited availability, but also because it has not been clearly demonstrated that treatment with Tamiflu, for example, would actually improve survival rates in clinical settings during a potential H5N1 pandemic. Nonetheless, given that the best pandemic response tool — vaccine — will be largely unavailable in the early going, governments can offer antiviral drug stockpiling as a tangible effort to protect their citizens.

Influenza as a Weapon

In the late 1990s, Congress authorized the Select Agent program to track the movement of certain bacteria and viruses that could potentially be used as bioterriorist weapons.[105] The program, which is administered by CDC and the U.S. Department of Agriculture, was expanded in statute following the anthrax attacks of 2001. An interagency working group determines which pathogens to place on the list of Select Agents. Once an organism is listed, those individuals and facilities working with it must be registered, undergo background investigations, and follow various guidelines in facility maintenance and management, shipping, recordkeeping and other practices. The list does not include common human strains of influenza, though it does include highly pathogenic strains of avian influenza, i.e., any strains which are shown to cause disease in commercial poultry. As such, H5N1 influenza is a covered pathogen. When scientists from the CDC and the Armed Forces Institute of Pathology recently re-created the 1918 pandemic flu virus, since it was a human influenza virus, it was not on the Select Agent list. It was subsequently added by HHS Secretary Leavitt on October 20, 2005.[106] Other flu strains which typically affect humans (rather than birds) remain unregulated at this time.

The matter of whether influenza viruses could be used deliberately as biological weapons has received recent attention in Congress. When asked about the possibility, CDC Director Julie Gerberding replied that "... we recognize that influenza has some of the important characteristics of an excellent threat agent. It's easily transmissible, it's relatively easy to produce and it's very easy to modify or engineer. So it does have characteristics that if a person was intent on modifying ..., it is not beyond our imagination to consider that beyond our preparedness efforts."[107] Dr. Gerberding also noted the natural behavior of the virus, which constantly shuffles its genes to produce new combinations, saying that "mother nature herself is a very effective terrorist.

REFERENCES

[1] World Organization for Animal Health (known by its French acronym, OIE), "Update on Avian Influenza in Animals in Asia (Type H5)," at [http://www.oie.int/downld/AVIAN%20INFLUENZA/A_AI-Asia.htm]. OIE is an intergovernmental organization of 167 nations and is not part of the United Nations system.

[2] World Health Organization, "Confirmed Human Cases of Avian Influenza A/(H5N1) ," as of Nov. 1, 2005, at [http://www.who.int/csr/disease/avian_influenza/country/en/].

[3] WHO, "Global Influenza Preparedness Plan: The Role of WHO and Recommendations for National Measures before and during Pandemics," 2005, (hereafter called the WHO pandemic plan), p. 3, at [http://www.who.int/csr/disease/influenza/pandemic/en/].

[4] Remarks of HHS Secretary Michael Leavitt on "Avian Flu," National Press Club, Oct. 27, 2005, CQ Transcriptions.

[5] David L. Heymann, *Control of Communicable Diseases Manual,* 18th ed., an official report of the American Public Health Association, 2004.

[6] CDC, Influenza home page, at [http://www.cdc.gov/flu/].

[7] WHO, "Avian Influenza — New Areas with Infection in Birds — Update 34," *Disease Outbreak News*, Oct. 13, 2005, at [http://www.who.int/csr/don/en/].

[8] Unless otherwise noted, information for this section is found in HHS, "Pandemics and Pandemic Scares in the 20th Century," Feb. 12, 2004, at [http://www.hhs.gov/nvpo/pandemics/flu3.htm#8].

[9] The U.S. population in 1918 was about one-third its current size, based on decennial census reports of more than 92 million in 1910, and more than 106 million in 1920. The U.S. population is currently almost 300 million. See [http://www.census.gov].

[10] Sources for this section are: Richard E. Neustadt and Harvey V. Fineberg, *The Swine Flu Affair,* a report to the Secretary of Health, Education and Welfare, June, 1978; and HHS Draft Pandemic Influenza Preparedness and Response Plan, Annex 11: "Lessons Learned from 1976 Swine Influenza Program," Aug. 2004. This incident is discussed further in a later section on vaccine liability and compensation issues.

[11] NIH, National Institute for Allergy and Infectious Diseases (NIAID), "NIAID Taps Chiron to Develop Vaccine Against H9N2 Avian Influenza," Aug. 17, 2004, at [http://www.nih.gov/news/].

[12] WHO, "Confirmed Human Cases of Avian Influenza A (H5N1)," at [http://www.who.int/csr/disease/avian_influenza/country/en/].

[13] WHO pandemic plan, p. 3.

[14] This phenomenon is often called a "cytokine storm," named after molecules in the immune system that are produced in excess. See C. Y. Cheung, et al., "Induction of Proinflammatory Cytokines in Human Macrophages by Influenza A (H5N1) Viruses: A Mechanism for the

Unusual Severity of Human Disease?" *Lancet*, vol. 360, Dec. 7, 2002, pp. 1831-1837; and Y. Guan, et al., "H5N1 Influenza: A Protean Pandemic Threat," *Proceedings of the National Academy of Sciences,* vol. 101(21), May 24, 2004, pp. 8156-8161.

[15] D. Kobasa, et al., "Enhanced Virulence of Influenza A Viruses with the Haemagglutinin of the 1918 Pandemic Virus," *Nature* vol. 431, Oct. 7, 2004, pp. 703-707.

[16] See Jeffery K. Taubenberger, et al., "Characterization of the 1918 Influenza Virus Polymerase Genes," *Nature*, vol. 437, pp. 889-893, Oct. 6, 2005; and Terrence M. Tumpey, et al., "Characterization of the Reconstructed 1918 Spanish Influenza Pandemic Virus," *Science,* vol. 310, Oct. 2005, pp. 77-80.

[17] Bosman, et al., "Final Analysis of Netherlands Avian Influenza Outbreaks Reveals Much Higher Levels of Transmission to Humans than Previously Thought," *Eurosurveillance Weekly,* vol. 10(1), Jan. 6, 2005, at [http://www.eurosurveillance.org/index-02.asp].

[18] WHO, "Avian Influenza A(H7) Human Infections in Canada," Apr. 5, 2004, at [http://www.who.int/csr/don/en/]; and CDC, "Avian Influenza Infections in Humans," Oct. 17, 2005, at [http://www.cdc.gov/flu/avian/gen-info/avian-flu-humans.htm].

[19] A.J. Hostetler and Calvin Trice, "Va. Worker May Have Caught Avian Flu," *Richmond Times-Dispatch,* Feb. 28, 2004.

[20] See CDC website on avian flu outbreaks in North America at [http://www.cdc.gov/flu/avian/outbreaks/us.htm].

[21] Comments of Klaus Stohr, in Keith Bradsher and Lawrence K. Altman, "WHO Official Says Deadly Pandemic Is Likely If the Asian Bird Flu Spreads Among People," *The New York Times*, Nov. 30, 2004.

[22] WHO, "Estimating the Impact of the Next Influenza Pandemic: Enhancing Preparedness," press release, Dec. 8, 2004, at [http://www.wpro.who.int/media_centre/press_releases/pr_20041209.htm].

[23] HHS "Pandemic Influenza Plan," Part 1: Strategic Plan, p. 18, Nov. 2005, at [http://www.pandemicflu.gov].

[24] Trust for America's Health (TFAH), *A Killer Flu?*, June 2005, at [http://healthyamericans.org/reports/flu/], applies a set of assumptions and ranges of severity to a CDC-developed computer model, FluAid 2.0, to generate death, hospitalization and outpatient rates based on populations with different age distributions. FluAid 2.0 is available at [http://www2a.cdc.gov/ od/fluaid/].

[25] M. I. Meltzer et al., "The Economic Impact of Pandemic Influenza in the United States: Priorities for Intervention," *Emerging Infectious Diseases*, vol. 5(5), Sept.-Oct. 1999.
[26] The World Bank Group, "Avian Flu: Economic Losses Could Top US$800 Billion," Nov. 8, 2005, at [http://www.worldbank.org/].
[27] Warwick J. McKibben, "SARS: Estimating the Economic Impacts," Institute of Medicine, Forum on Microbial Threats, Workshop, "Learning from SARS: Preparing for the Next Disease Outbreak," Sept. 30, 2003, at [http://www.iom.edu/event.asp?id=14647].
[28] Alison Appelbe, "Canada Blames Media Hype for SARS Economic Impact," CNSNews.com, Apr. 25, 2003.
[29] WHO pandemic plan.
[30] HHS, *Draft Pandemic Influenza Preparedness and Response Plan*, Aug. 26, 2004, at [http://www.hhs.gov/nvpo/pandemicplan/index.html].
[31] See, for example, Association of State and Territorial Health Officials (ASTHO), comments on the HHS National Pandemic Influenza Preparedness and Response Plan, Oct. 25, 2004, at [http://www.astho.org/pubs/ASTHOCommentsonPandemicFluPlan.pdf], hereafter cited as ASTHO comments regarding HHS plan. Additional comments are at HHS, "Public Comments to the Pandemic Influenza Preparedness and Response Plan," at [http://www.hhs.gov/nvpo/pandemicplan/comments062005.html].
[32] White House Homeland Security Council, *National Strategy for Pandemic Influenza,* Nov. 1, 2005, at [http://www.pandemicflu.gov/].
[33] See White House Office of Management and Budget, Estimate No. 15, Nov. 1, 2005, at [http://www.whitehouse.gov/omb/budget/amendments/supplemental_11_01_05.pdf].
[34] HHS, "HHS Pandemic Influenza Plan," Nov. 2005, at [http://www.pandemicflu.gov].
[35] Though the plan includes specific tiers of priority groups, and estimates of the number of people in each group, the designations may be modified in light of the actual behavior of a pandemic flu strain. For example, if atypical groups such as healthy young people were found to be at increased risk of severe illness, the tiers could be adjusted accordingly.
[36] Department of Defense, "Pandemic Influenza Preparation and Response Planning Guidance," Sept. 15, 2004, at [http://www.geis.fhp.osd.mil/GEIS/SurveillanceActivities/Influenza/fluPolicy.asp].

[37] See [http://deploymentlink.osd.mil/medical/medical_issues/immun/avian_flu.shtml].

[38] See DOD Global Emerging Infections System at [http://www.geis.fhp.osd.mil/aboutGEIS.asp] VA, "Pandemic Flu Planning and the Department of Veterans Affairs: Overview," Oct., 2005, at [http://vhaaidsinfo.cio.med.va.gov/flu/documents/Avian_Flu_Public_final.pdf], found on the VA influenza page at [http://vhaaidsinfo.cio.med.va.gov/flu/pandemicflu.htm].

[39] According to cooperative agreement guidance for FY2004 funds, states were required to submit pandemic plans along with their applications for FY2005 funds. See CDC, "Cooperative Agreement Guidance for Public Health Emergency Preparedness," Program Announcement AA154, May 13, 2005, at [http://www.bt.cdc.gov/planning/guidance05/].

[40] Communication with Michael Craig, CDC Policy Analyst, Nov. 1, 2005. According to the Public Health Service Act, the District of Columbia is considered a state for purposes of preparedness funding and requirements.

[41] Council of State and Territorial Epidemiologists, state pandemic influenza plans, at [http://www.cste.org/specialprojects/Influenzaplans/StateMap.asp]. CDC is not involved in maintaining this site and cannot confirm whether plans available here are the same versions as those submitted to the agency.

[42] CDC, "Pandemic Influenza: A Planning Guide for State and Local Officials (Draft 2.1)," undated document.

[43] ASTHO, "Nature's Terrorist Attack: Pandemic Influenza, Preparedness Planning for State Health Officials," Nov. 2002, at [http://www.astho.org/ pubs/Pandemic%20Influenza.pdf].

[44] See DHS, *National Response Plan*, Dec. 2004, hereafter called the NRP, at [http://www.dhs.gov/dhspublic/display?theme=14andcontent=4264], and CRS Report RL32803, *The National Preparedness System: Issues in the 109th Congress*, by Keith Bea.

[45] Testimony of Dr. Jeffrey Runge, Chief Medical Officer, DHS, before the House Homeland Security Committee, Subcommittee on Management, Integration, and Oversight, hearing on "Role of the Chief Medical Officer," Oct. 27, 2005, 109th Congress, 1st Sess.

[46] For more information on ESF#8, see CRS Report RL33096, *2005 Gulf Coast Hurricanes: The Public Health and Medical Response*, by Sarah A. Lister.

[47] See CRS Report RS21227, *The Emergency Management Assistance Compact (EMAC): An Overview*, by Keith Bea.

[48] The administration's emergency supplemental budget request for pandemic flu, submitted to Congress on Nov. 1, 2005, would provide $47.3 million to DHS, for several activities including the development of pandemic response exercises.

[49] The term *police powers* derives from the 10th Amendment to the Constitution, which reserves to the states those rights and powers not delegated to the United States. Historically these have been interpreted to include authority over the welfare, safety, health, and morals of the public.

[50] A public health emergency was declared in several states affected by Hurricane Katrina. See CRS Report RL33096, *2005 Gulf Coast Hurricanes: The Public Health and Medical Response*, by Sarah A. Lister.

[51] For a discussion of the exercise of federal and state authorities in response to the recent shortage of influenza vaccine, see CRS Report RL32655, *Influenza Vaccine Shortages and Implications*, by Sarah A. Lister and Erin D. Williams.

[52] NRP, Biological Incident Annex, p. BIO-1.

[53] See CRS Report RL33053, *Federal Stafford Act Disaster Assistance: Presidential Declarations, Eligible Activities, and Funding*, by Keith Bea.

[54] See comments of New Jersey Governor Richard Codey in Rick Hepp, "Jersey Officials Identify Holes in Response Plan," *The Star-Ledger,* Apr. 9, 2005.

[55] NRP, Catastrophic Incident Annex, p. CAT-1.

[56] Chris Strohm, "DHS Failed to Use Catastrophe Response Plan in Katrina's Wake," *GovExec.com*, Oct. 18, 2005.

[57] Zack Phillips, "DHS Catastrophe Plan Incomplete, Congressmen Say," *CQ Homeland Security,* Nov. 1, 2005.

[58] CDC, "Overview of Influenza Surveillance in the United States," Feb. 2, 2005, at [http://www.cdc.gov/flu/weekly/pdf/flu-surveillance-overview.pdf].

[59] CDC, "Health Updates on Avian Influenza," Feb. 4, 2005 and previous, at [http://www.cdc.gov/flu/avian/professional/updates.htm].

[60] CDC, "Key Facts About Avian Influenza (Bird Flu) and Avian Influenza A (H5N1) Virus," Oct. 25, 2005, at [http://www.cdc.gov/flu/avian/gen-info/facts.htm]. If a state were to identify H5 strains of

influenza, the specimens would then be referred to CDC to determine if they were H5N1.

[61] See CRS Report RL31333, *Federal and State Isolation and Quarantine Authority*, by Angie A. Welborn.

[62] See Executive Order: "Amendment to E.O. 13295 Relating to Certain Influenza Viruses and Quarantinable Communicable Diseases," Apr. 1, 2005, at [http://www.whitehouse.gov/ news/releases/2005/04/20050401-6.html]; and CDC, "Questions and Answers on the Executive Order Adding Potentially Pandemic Influenza Viruses to the List of Quarantinable Diseases," Apr. 11, 2005, at [http://www.cdc.gov/ncidod/dq/qa_influenza_amendment_ to_eo_13295.htm].

[63] See CDC Division of Global Migration and Quarantine home page at [http://www.cdc.gov/ncidod/dq/index.htm].

[64] Press conference with President George Bush, Federal News Service transcript, Oct. 4, 2005.

[65] CRS Report RL31615, *Homeland Security: The Department of Defense's Role*, by Steve Bowman.

[66] NRP, "Defense Support of Civil Authorities," pp. 41 ff.

[67] CRS Report RS22266 , *The Use of Federal Troops for Disaster Assistance: Legal Issues*, by Jennifer K. Elsea.

[68] Information provided by Dr. Dale Smith, medical historian, Uniformed Services University of the Health Sciences, Bethesda, Maryland, Oct. 13, 2005.

[69] Mark Mazzetti, "Military Sees Limits to Role in U.S. Disasters; A Defense official says 'catastrophic' events, including a pandemic, would be the threshold," Oct. 13, 2005.

[70] Christophe Fraser, et al., "Factors that Make an Infectious Disease Outbreak Controllable," *Proceedings of the National Academy of Sciences,* vol. 101(16), pp. 6146-6151, Apr. 20, 2004, at [http://www.pnas.org/cgi/reprint/101/16/6146].

[71] See, for example, Brian Friel, "Law In The Time Of Cholera," *National Journal,* Oct. 21, 2005.

[72] Charles M. Helms, NVAC Chairman, letter to HHS Acting Assistant Secretary for Health Cristina V. Beato, on NVAC recommendations regarding priority use of vaccine and antiviral drugs during an influenza pandemic, Aug. 10, 2005, at [http://www.hhs.gov/nvpo/nvac /documents/chairletter.pdf].

[73] For more information on rationing of scarce health resources, see the section on Strategies for Rationing in CRS Report RL32655, *Influenza*

Vaccine Shortages and Implications, by Sarah A. Lister and Erin D. Williams.

[74] Further discussion of flu vaccine production is available in CRS Report RL32655, *Influenza Vaccine Shortages and Implications*, by Sarah A. Lister and Erin D. Williams.

[75] Recently, WHO and some countries have considered stockpiling small amounts of a prototype H5N1 vaccine. There is concern that if H5N1 became a pandemic strain, it might change sufficiently that "pre-pandemic" vaccine may not protect.

[76] David S. Fedson, "Preparing for Pandemic Vaccination: An International Policy Agenda for Vaccine Development," *Journal of Public Health Policy,* Vol. 26, pp. 4-29, 2005, (hereafter called Fedson article), at [http://www.palgrave-journals.com/jphp/fedson.pdf].

[77] The company does not use capital letters in its name.

[78] See White House Office of Management and Budget, Estimate No. 15, Nov. 1, 2005, at [http://www.whitehouse.gov/omb/budget /amendments/supplemental_11_01_05.pdf].

[79] Testimony of HHS Secretary Michael Leavitt before the Senate Committee on Appropriations, Subcommittee on Labor, Health and Human Services, Education, and Related Agencies, hearing on "Pandemic Flu," Nov. 2, 2005, 109th Congress, 1st Sess.

[80] See Fedson article. The author also comments that the United States has been ahead of other countries in providing public funding to support the development of prototype pandemic vaccines.

[81] Presentation of Jesse L. Goodman, Director, FDA Center for Biologics Evaluation and Research, "Meeting the Challenge of Pandemic Vaccine Preparedness: An FDA Perspective," at the Institute of Medicine Symposium on Pandemic Influenza Research, Apr. 5, 2005, at [http://www.iom.edu/project.asp?id=25218]. See also Jennifer Corbett Dooren, "FDA Aims to Approve New Flu Treatments in Weeks," Dow Jones News Service, Nov. 4, 2005.

[82] Reverse genetics is a technique to modify viruses so they can be grown more easily for vaccine production. Cell culture is a streamlined method of growing large amounts of virus. Both techniques are explained in greater detail in CRS Report RL32655, *Influenza Vaccine Shortages and Implications*, by Sarah A. Lister and Erin D. Williams.

[83] See NIH: National Institute of Allergy and Infectious Diseases influenza page at [http://www.niaid.nih.gov/dmid/influenza/]; and

Pandemic Influenza Preparedness Program page, at [http://www.niaid.nih.gov/dmid/influenza/panintro.htm].

[84] FDA, "Emergency Use Authorization of Medical Products," draft guidance, not for implementation, June 2005, at [http://www.fda.gov/cber/gdlns/emeruse.pdf]. The authority to declare an emergency authorizing this use is also provided in P.L. 108-276, and is somewhat broader than the HHS Secretary's public health emergency authority.

[85] FDA, "Authorization of Emergency Use of Anthrax Vaccine Adsorbed for Prevention of Inhalation Anthrax by Individuals at Heightened Risk of Exposure Due to Attack With Anthrax; Availability," 70 *Federal Register* 5452, Feb. 2, 2005.

[86] For more information, see the National Vaccine Injury Compensation Program Home Page at [http://www.hrsa.gov/osp/vicp/INDEX.HTM].

[87] See CRS Report RL31960, *Smallpox Vaccine Injury Compensation*, by Susan Thaul.

[88] Sources for this section are: Richard E. Neustadt and Harvey V. Fineberg, *The Swine Flu Affair,* a report to the Secretary of Health, Education and Welfare, June, 1978; and HHS Draft Pandemic Influenza Preparedness and Response Plan, Annex 11: "Lessons Learned from the 1976 Swine Influenza Program," Aug. 2004.

[89] U.S. Department of Justice, Civil Division, Torts Branch, "Swine Flu Statistics," Jan. 3, 1991. Overall, 4,179 claims were filed under the act. Not all claims were resolved administratively, and 1,604 claimants proceeded to file suit.

[90] Letter from HHS Secretary Michael Leavitt to House Speaker Dennis Hastert regarding the draft bill,"Pandemic Flu Countermeasure Liability Protection Act," Nov. 1, 2005.

[91] See CRS Report RL32051: *Innovation and Intellectual Property Issues in Homeland Security*, by John R. Thomas. This authority is based in existing law and does not require an emergency declaration or other special circumstance.

[92] See Fedson article.

[93] Ibid.

[94] See CDC, antivirals for influenza at [http://www.cdc.gov/flu/professionals/treatment/].

[95] See, for example, Fu Jing, "Misuse of antiviral on poultry must stop," *China Daily*, June 21, 2005, at [http://www.chinadaily.com.cn/english/doc/2005-06/21/content_453023.htm].

[96] Q. Mai Le, "Avian Flu: Isolation of Drug-resistant H5N1 Virus," *Nature* 437, 1108 Oct, 20, 2005; and Luciana L. Borio and John G. Bartlett, "Isolation of H5N1 Influenza Virus Resistant to Oseltamivir," *Clinician's Biosecurity Network Weekly Bulletin*, Oct. 18, 2005.

[97] Statement of George B. Abercrombie, President and Chief Executive Officer, Hoffman-La Roche Inc., before the Committee on Government Reform, U.S. House of Representatives, hearing on "The Next Flu Pandemic: Evaluating U.S. Readiness," June 30, 2005, 109th Congress, 1st Sess.

[98] Roche, "Tamiflu Facts and Figures," Oct. 27, 2005, at [http://www.roche.com/home.html].

[99] See also, Andrew Pollack, "Is a Bird Flu Drug Really So Vexing?" *The New York Times,* Nov. 5, 2005.

[100] See "Shipments of Flu Drug Suspended: Tamiflu Maker Moves to Foil Hoarding, Meet Winter Demand," *The Washington Post,* Oct. 28, 2005.

[101] Testimony of CDC Director Julie Gerberding before the Senate Committee on Foreign Relations, hearing on "Avian Influenza — Are We Prepared?" Nov. 9, 2005, 109th Congress, 1st Sess.

[102] The NVAC had recommended stockpiling of antiviral drugs sufficient to treat 13% of the population as the minimal requirement, and that amounts sufficient for 45% of the population would be optimal.

[103] Testimony of HHS Secretary Michael Leavitt before the Senate Committee on Appropriations, Subcommittee on Labor, Health and Human Services, Education, and Related Agencies, hearing on "Pandemic Flu," Nov. 2, 2005, 109th Congress, 1st Sess.

[104] See Gardiner Harris, "Administration's Flu Plan Gets Mixed Reception in Congress," *The New York Times,* Nov. 3, 2005.

[105] For more information, see the CDC Select Agent program page at [http://www.cdc.gov/od/sap] and CRS Report RL31719, *An Overview of the U.S. Public Health System in the Context of Emergency Preparedness*, by Sarah A. Lister.

[106] CDC, "Possession, Use, and Transfer of Select Agents and Toxins - Reconstructed Replication Competent Forms of the 1918 Pandemic Influenza Virus Containing Any Portion of the Coding Regions of All Eight Gene Segments," 70 *Federal Register* 61047, Oct. 20, 2005.

[107] Testimony of CDC Director Julie Gerberding before the House Committee on Homeland Security, Subcommittee on Prevention of Nuclear and Biological Attacks, hearing on "National Biodefense Strategy," July 28, 2005, 109th Congress, 1st Sess.

In: Global Spread of the Avian Flu… ISBN 1-60021-011-2
Editors: M.R. Bethe, pp. 121-138

Chapter 5

NATIONAL STRATEGY FOR PANDEMIC INFLUENZA

Homeland Security Council

My fellow Americans,

Once again, nature has presented us with a daunting challenge: the possibility of an influenza pandemic.

Most of us are accustomed to seasonal influenza, or "the flu," a viral infection that continues to be a significant public health challenge. From time to time, changes in the influenza virus result in a new strain to which people have never been exposed. These new strains have the potential to sweep the globe, causing millions of illnesses, in what is called a pandemic.

A new strain of influenza virus has been found in birds in Asia, and has shown that it can infect humans. If this virus undergoes further change, it could very well result in the next human pandemic.

We have an opportunity to prepare ourselves, our Nation, and our world to fight this potentially devastating outbreak of infectious disease.

The *National Strategy for Pandemic Influenza* presents our approach to address the threat of pandemic influenza, whether it results from the strain currently in birds in Asia or another influenza virus. It outlines how we intend to prepare, detect, and respond to a pandemic. It also outlines the important roles to be played not only by the Federal government, but also by State and local governments, private industry, our international partners, and most importantly individual citizens, including you and your families.

While your government will do much to prepare for a pandemic, individual action and individual responsibility are necessary for the success of any measures. Not only should you take action to protect yourself and your families, you should also take action to prevent the spread of influenza if you or anyone in your family becomes ill.

Together we will confront this emerging threat and together, as Americans, we will be prepared to protect our families, our communities, this great Nation, and our world.

GEORGE W. BUSH,
THE WHITE HOUSE
November 1, 2005

INTRODUCTION

Although remarkable advances have been made in science and medicine during the past century, we are constantly reminded that we live in a universe of microbes - viruses, bacteria, protozoa and fungi that are forever changing and adapting themselves to the human host and the defenses that humans create.

Influenza viruses are notable for their resilience and adaptability. While science has been able to develop highly effective vaccines and treatments for many infectious diseases that threaten public health, acquiring these tools is an ongoing challenge with the influenza virus. Changes in the genetic makeup of the virus require us to develop new vaccines on an annual basis and forecast which strains are likely to predominate.

As a result, and despite annual vaccinations, the U.S. faces a burden of influenza that results in approximately 36,000 deaths and more than 200,000 hospitalizations each year. In addition to this human toll, influenza is annually responsible for a total cost of over $10 billion in the U.S.

A pandemic, or worldwide outbreak of a new influenza virus, could dwarf this impact by overwhelming our health and medical capabilities, potentially resulting in hundreds of thousands of deaths, millions of hospitalizations, and hundreds of billions of dollars in direct and indirect costs. This *Strategy* will guide our preparedness and response activities to mitigate that impact.

THE PANDEMIC THREAT

Pandemics happen when a novel influenza virus emerges that infects and can be efficiently transmitted between humans. Animals are the most likely reservoir for these emerging viruses; avian viruses played a role in the last three influenza pandemics. Two of these pandemic-causing viruses remain in circulation and are responsible for the majority of influenza cases each year.

Pandemics have occurred intermittently over centuries. The last three pandemics, in 1918, 1957 and 1968, killed approximately 40 million, 2 million and 1 million people worldwide, respectively. Although the timing cannot be predicted, history and science suggest that we will face one or more pandemics in this century.

The current pandemic threat stems from an unprecedented outbreak of avian influenza in Asia and Europe, caused by the H5N1 strain of the Influenza A virus. To date, the virus has infected birds in 16 countries and has resulted in the deaths, through illness and culling, of approximately 200 million birds across Asia. While traditional control measures have been attempted, the virus is now endemic in Southeast Asia, present in long-range migratory birds, and unlikely to be eradicated soon.

A notable and worrisome feature of the H5N1 virus is its ability to infect a wide range of hosts, including birds and humans. As of the date of this document, the virus is known to have infected 121 people in four countries, resulting in 62 deaths over the past two years. Although the virus has not yet shown an ability to transmit efficiently between humans, as is seen with the annual influenza virus, there is concern that it will acquire this capability through genetic mutation or exchange of genetic material with a human influenza virus.

It is impossible to know whether the currently circulating H5N1 virus will cause a human pandemic. The widespread nature of H5N1 in birds and the likelihood of mutations over time raise our concerns that the virus will become transmissible between humans, with potentially catastrophic consequences. If this does not happen with the current H5N1 strain, history suggests that a different influenza virus will emerge and result in the next pandemic.

THE NATIONAL STRATEGY FOR PANDEMIC INFLUENZA

Preparing for a pandemic requires the leveraging of all instruments of national power, and coordinated action by all segments of government and society. Influenza viruses do not respect the distinctions of race, sex, age, profession or nationality, and are not constrained by geographic boundaries. The next pandemic is likely to come in waves, each lasting months, and pass through communities of all size across the nation and world. While a pandemic will not damage power lines, banks or computer networks, it will ultimately threaten all critical infrastructure by removing essential personnel from the workplace for weeks or months.

This makes a pandemic a unique circumstance necessitating a strategy that extends well beyond health and medical boundaries, to include the sustainment of critical infrastructure, private-sector activities, the movement of goods and services across the nation and the globe, and economic and security considerations. The uncertainties associated with influenza viruses require that our *Strategy* be versatile, to ensure that we are prepared for any virus with pandemic potential, as well as the annual burden of influenza that we know we will face.

The *National Strategy for Pandemic Influenza* guides our preparedness and response to an influenza pandemic, with the intent of (1) stopping, slowing or otherwise limiting the spread of a pandemic to the United States; (2) limiting the domestic spread of a pandemic, and mitigating disease, suffering and death; and (3) sustaining infrastructure and mitigating impact to the economy and the functioning of society.

The *Strategy* will provide a framework for future U.S. Government planning efforts that is consistent with *The National Security Strategy* and the *National Strategy for Homeland Security*. It recognizes that preparing for and responding to a pandemic cannot be viewed as a purely federal responsibility, and that the nation must have a system of plans at all levels of government and in all sectors outside of government that can be integrated to address the pandemic threat. It is guided by the following principles:

- The federal government will use all instruments of national power to address the pandemic threat.
- States and communities should have credible pandemic preparedness plans to respond to an outbreak within their jurisdictions.

- The private sector should play an integral role in preparedness before a pandemic begins, and should be part of the national response.
- Individual citizens should be prepared for an influenza pandemic, and be educated about individual responsibility to limit the spread of infection if they or their family members become ill.
- Global partnerships will be leveraged to address the pandemic threat.

PILLARS OF THE NATIONAL STRATEGY

Our Strategy addresses the full spectrum of events that link a farmyard overseas to a living room in America. While the circumstances that connect these environments are very different, our strategic principles remain relevant. The pillars of our Strategy are:

- **Preparedness and Communication**: Activities that should be undertaken before a pandemic to ensure preparedness, and the communication of roles and responsibilities to all levels of government, segments of society and individuals.
- **Surveillance and Detection**: Domestic and international systems that provide continuous "situational awareness," to ensure the earliest warning possible to protect the population.
- **Response and Containment**: Actions to limit the spread of the outbreak and to mitigate the health, social and economic impacts of a pandemic.

IMPLEMENTATION OF THE *NATIONAL STRATEGY*

This Strategy reflects the federal government's approach to the pandemic threat. While it provides strategic direction for the Departments and Agencies of the U.S. Government, it does not attempt to catalogue and assign all federal responsibilities. The implementation of this Strategy and specific responsibilities will be described separately.

PILLAR ONE: PREPAREDNESS AND COMMUNICATION

Preparedness is the underpinning of the entire spectrum of activities, including surveillance, detection, containment and response efforts. We will support pandemic planning efforts, and clearly communicate expectations to individuals, communities and governments, whether overseas or in the United States, recognizing that all share the responsibility to limit the spread of infection in order to protect populations beyond their borders.

Planning for a Pandemic

To enhance preparedness, we will:

- Develop federal implementation plans to support this *Strategy*, to include all components of the U.S. government and to address the full range of consequences of a pandemic, including human and animal health, security, transportation, economic, trade and infrastructure considerations.
- Work through multilateral health organizations such as the World Health Organization (WHO), Food and Agriculture Organization (FAO), World Organization for Animal Health (OIE) and regional organizations such as the Asia-Pacific Economic Cooperation (APEC) forum, as well as through bilateral and multilateral contacts to:
  - Support the development and exercising of avian and pandemic response plans;
  - Expand in-country medical, veterinary and scientific capacity to respond to an outbreak; and
  - Educate populations at home and abroad about high-risk practices that increase the likelihood of virus transmission between species.
- Continue to work with states and localities to:
  - Establish and exercise pandemic response plans;
  - Develop medical and veterinary surge capacity plans; and
  - Integrate non-health sectors, including the private sector and critical infrastructure entities, in these planning efforts.
- Build upon existing domestic mechanisms to rapidly recruit and deploy large numbers of health, medical and veterinary providers

within or across jurisdictions to match medical requirements with capabilities.

Communicating Expectations and Responsibilities

A critical element of pandemic planning is ensuring that people and entities not accustomed to responding to health crises understand the actions and priorities required to prepare for and respond to a pandemic. Those groups include political leadership at all levels of government, nonhealth components of government and members of the private sector. Essential planning also includes the coordination of efforts between human and animal health authorities. In order to accomplish this, we will:

- Work to ensure clear, effective and coordinated risk communication, domestically and internationally, before and during a pandemic. This includes identifying credible spokespersons at all levels of government to effectively coordinate and communicate helpful, informative messages in a timely manner.
- Provide guidance to the private sector and critical infrastructure entities on their role in the pandemic response, and considerations necessary to maintain essential services and operations despite significant and sustained worker absenteeism.
- Provide guidance to individuals on infection control behaviors they should adopt pre-pandemic, and the specific actions they will need to take during a severe influenza season or pandemic, such as self-isolation and protection of others if they themselves contract influenza.
- Provide guidance and support to poultry, swine and related industries on their role in responding to an outbreak of avian influenza, including ensuring the protection of animal workers and initiating or strengthening public education campaigns to minimize the risks of infection from animal products.

Producing and Stockpiling Vaccines, Antivirals and Medical Material

In combination with traditional public health measures, vaccines and antiviral drugs form the foundation of our infection control strategy.

Vaccination is the most important element of this strategy, but we acknowledge that a two-pronged strategy incorporating both vaccines and antivirals is essential. To establish production capacity and stockpiles in support of our containment and response strategies, we will:

- Encourage nations to develop production capacity and stockpiles to support their response needs, to include pooling of efforts to create regional capacity.
- Encourage and subsidize the development of state-based antiviral stockpiles to support response activities.
- Ensure that our national stockpile and stockpiles based in states and communities are properly configured to respond to the diversity of medical requirements presented by a pandemic, including personal protective equipment, antibiotics and general supplies.
- Establish domestic production capacity and stockpiles of countermeasures to ensure:
  - Sufficient vaccine to vaccinate front-line personnel and at-risk populations, including military personnel;
  - Sufficient vaccine to vaccinate the entire U.S. population within six months of the emergence of a virus with pandemic potential; and
  - Antiviral treatment for those who contract a pandemic strain of influenza.
- Facilitate appropriate coordination of efforts across the vaccine manufacturing sector.
- Address regulatory and other legal barriers to the expansion of our domestic vaccine production capacity.
- Expand the public health recommendations for domestic seasonal influenza vaccination and encourage the same practice internationally.
- Expand the domestic supply of avian influenza vaccine to control a domestic outbreak of avian influenza in bird populations.

Establishing Distribution Plans for Vaccines and Antivirals

It is essential that we prioritize the allocation of countermeasures (vaccines and antivirals) that are in limited supply and define effective distribution modalities during a pandemic. We will:

- Develop credible countermeasure distribution mechanisms for vaccine and antiviral agents prior to and during a pandemic.
- Prioritize countermeasure allocation before an outbreak, and update this prioritization immediately after the outbreak begins based on the at-risk populations, available supplies and the characteristics of the virus.

Advancing Scientific Knowledge and Accelerating Development

Research and development of vaccines, antivirals, adjuvants and diagnostics represents our best defense against a pandemic. To realize our goal of nextgeneration countermeasures against influenza, we must make significant and targeted investments in promising technologies. We will:

- Ensure that there is maximal sharing of scientific information about influenza viruses between governments, scientific entities and the private sector.
- Work with our international partners to ensure that we are all leveraging the most advanced technological approaches available for vaccine production.
- Accelerate the development of cell culture technology for influenza vaccine production and establish a domestic production base to support vaccination demands.
- Use novel investment strategies to advance the development of nextgeneration influenza diagnostics and countermeasures, including new antivirals, vaccines, adjuvant technologies, and countermeasures that provide protection across multiple strains and seasons of the influenza virus.

Pillar Two: Surveillance and Detection

Early warning of a pandemic and our ability to closely track the spread of avian influenza outbreak is critical to being able to rapidly employ resources to contain the spread of the virus. An effective surveillance and detection system will save lives by allowing us to activate our response plans before the arrival of a pandemic virus to the U.S., activate additional surveillance systems and initiate vaccine production and administration.

Ensuring Rapid Reporting of Outbreaks

To support our need for "situational awareness," both domestically and internationally, we will:

- Work through the International Partnership on Avian and Pandemic Influenza, as well as through other political and diplomatic channels such as the United Nations and the Asia- Pacific Economic Cooperation forum, to ensure transparency, scientific cooperation and rapid reporting of avian and human influenza cases.
- Support the development of the proper scientific and epidemiologic expertise in affected regions to ensure early recognition of changes in the pattern of avian or human outbreaks.
- Support the development and sustainment of sufficient U.S. and host nation laboratory capacity and diagnostic reagents in affected regions and domestically, to provide rapid confirmation of cases in animals or humans.
- Advance mechanisms for "real-time" clinical surveillance in domestic acute care settings such as emergency departments, intensive care units and laboratories to provide local, state and federal public health officials with continuous awareness of the profile of illness in communities, and leverage all federal medical capabilities, both domestic and international, in support of this objective.
- Develop and deploy rapid diagnostics with greater sensitivity and reproducibility to allow onsite diagnosis of pandemic strains of influenza at home and abroad, in animals and humans, to facilitate early warning, outbreak control and targeting of antiviral therapy.
- Expand our domestic livestock and wildlife surveillance activities to ensure early warning of the spread of an outbreak to our shores.

Using Surveillance to Limit Spread

Although influenza does not respect geographic or political borders, entry to and egress from affected areas represent opportunities to control or at the very least slow the spread of infection. In parallel to our containment measures, we will:

- Develop mechanisms to rapidly share information on travelers who may be carrying or may have been exposed to a pandemic strain of influenza, for the purposes of contact tracing and outbreak investigation.
- Develop and exercise mechanisms to provide active and passive surveillance during an outbreak, both within and beyond our borders.
- Expand and enhance mechanisms for screening and monitoring animals that may harbor viruses with pandemic potential.
- Develop screening and monitoring mechanisms and agreements to appropriately control travel and shipping of potentially infected products to and from affected regions if necessary, and to protect unaffected populations.

PILLAR THREE: RESPONSE AND CONTAINMENT

We recognize that a virus with pandemic potential anywhere represents a risk to populations everywhere. Once health authorities have signaled sustained and efficient human-to-human spread of the virus has occurred, a cascade of response mechanisms will be initiated, from the site of the documented transmission to locations around the globe.

Containing Outbreaks

The most effective way to protect the American population is to contain an outbreak beyond the borders of the U.S. While we work to prevent a pandemic from reaching our shores, we recognize that slowing or limiting the spread of the outbreak is a more realistic outcome and can save many lives. In support of our containment strategy, we will:

- Work through the International Partnership to develop a coalition of strong partners to coordinate actions to limit the spread of a virus with pandemic potential beyond the location where it is first recognized in order to protect U.S. interests abroad.
- Where appropriate, offer and coordinate assistance from the United States and other members of the International Partnership.

- Encourage all levels of government, domestically and globally, to take appropriate and lawful action to contain an outbreak within the borders of their community, province, state or nation.
- Where appropriate, use governmental authorities to limit non-essential movement of people, goods and services into and out of areas where an outbreak occurs.
- Provide guidance to all levels of government on the range of options for infection-control and containment, including those circumstances where social distancing measures, limitations on gatherings, or quarantine authority may be an appropriate public health intervention.
- Emphasize the roles and responsibilities of the individual in preventing the spread of an outbreak, and the risk to others if infection-control practices are not followed.
- Provide guidance for states, localities and industry on best practices to prevent the spread of avian influenza in commercial, domestic and wild birds, and other animals.

Leveraging National Medical and Public Health Surge Capacity

Rather than generating a focal point of casualties, the medical burden of a pandemic is likely to be distributed in communities across the nation for an extended period of time. In order to save lives and limit suffering, we will:

- Implement state and local public health and medical surge plans, and leverage all federal medical facilities, personnel and response capabilities to support the national surge requirement.
- Activate plans to distribute medical countermeasures, including non-medical equipment and other material, from the Strategic National Stockpile and other distribution centers to federal, state and local authorities.
- Address barriers to the flow of public health, medical and veterinary personnel across state and local jurisdictions to meet local shortfalls in public health, medical and veterinary capacity.
- Determine the spectrum of public health, medical and veterinary surge capacity activities that the U.S. military and other government entities may be able to support during a pandemic, contingent upon

primary mission requirements, and develop mechanisms to activate them.

Sustaining Infrastructure, Essential Services and the Economy

Movement of essential personnel, goods and services, and maintenance of critical infrastructure are necessary during an event that spans months in any given community. The private sector and critical infrastructure entities must respond in a manner that allows them to maintain the essential elements of their operations for a prolonged period of time, in order to prevent severe disruption of life in our communities. To ensure this, we will:

- Encourage the development of coordination mechanisms across American industries to support the above activities during a pandemic.
- Provide guidance to activate contingency plans to ensure that personnel are protected, that the delivery of essential goods and services is maintained, and that sectors remain functional despite significant and sustained worker absenteeism.
- Determine the spectrum of infrastructure-sustainment activities that the U.S. military and other government entities may be able to support during a pandemic, contingent upon primary mission requirements, and develop mechanisms to activate them.

Ensuring Effective Risk Communication

Effective risk communication is essential to inform the public and mitigate panic. We will:

- Ensure that timely, clear, coordinated messages are delivered to the American public from trained spokespersons at all levels of government and assist the governments of affected nations to do the same.
- Work with state and local governments to develop guidelines to assure the public of the safety of the food supply and mitigate the risk of exposure from wildlife.

Roles and Responsibilities

Because of its unique nature, responsibility for preparedness and response to a pandemic extends across all levels of government and all segments of society. No single entity alone can prevent or mitigate the impact of a pandemic.

The Federal Government

While the Federal government plays a critical role in elements of preparedness and response to a pandemic, the success of these measures is predicated on actions taken at the individual level and in states and communities. Federal responsibilities include the following:

- Advancing international preparedness, surveillance, response and containment activities.
- Supporting the establishment of countermeasure stockpiles and production capacity by:
  - Facilitating the development of sufficient domestic production capacity for vaccines, antivirals, diagnostics and personal protective equipment to support domestic needs, and encouraging the development of production capacity around the world;
  - Advancing the science necessary to produce effective vaccines, therapeutics and diagnostics; and
  - Stockpiling and coordinating the distribution of necessary countermeasures, in concert with states and other entities.
- Ensuring that federal departments and agencies, including federal health care systems, have developed and exercised preparedness and response plans that take into account the potential impact of a pandemic on the federal workforce, and are configured to support state, local and private sector efforts as appropriate.
- Facilitating state and local planning through funding and guidance.
- Providing guidance to the private sector and public on preparedness and response planning, in conjunction with states and communities.

Lead departments have been identified for the medical response (Department of Health and Human Services), veterinary response

(Department of Agriculture), international activities (Department of State) and the overall domestic incident management and Federal coordination (Department of Homeland Security). Each department is responsible for coordination of all efforts within its authorized mission, and departments are responsible for developing plans to implement this *Strategy*.

States and Localities

Our communities are on the front lines of a pandemic and will face many challenges in maintaining continuity of society in the face of widespread illness and increased demand on most essential government services. State and local responsibilities include the following:

- Ensuring that all reasonable measures are taken to limit the spread of an outbreak within and beyond the community's borders.
- Establishing comprehensive and credible preparedness and response plans that are exercised on a regular basis.
- Integrating non-health entities in the planning for a pandemic, including law enforcement, utilities, city services and political leadership.
- Establishing state and community-based stockpiles and distribution systems to support a comprehensive pandemic response.
- Identifying key spokespersons for the community, ensuring that they are educated in risk communication, and have coordinated crisis communications plans.
- Providing public education campaigns on pandemic influenza and public and private interventions.

The Private Sector and Critical Infrastructure Entities

The private sector represents an essential pillar of our society because of the essential goods and services that it provides. Moreover, it touches the majority of our population on a daily basis, through an employer-employee or vendor-customer relationship. For these reasons, it is essential that the U.S. private sector be engaged in all preparedness and response activities for a pandemic.

Critical infrastructure entities also must be engaged in planning for a pandemic because of our society's dependence upon their services. Both the private sector and critical infrastructure entities represent essential underpinnings for the functioning of American society. Responsibilities of the U.S. private sector and critical infrastructure entities include the following:

- Establishing an ethic of infection control in the workplace that is reinforced during the annual influenza season, to include, if possible, options for working offsite while ill, systems to reduce infection transmission, and worker education.
- Establishing contingency systems to maintain delivery of essential goods and services during times of significant and sustained worker absenteeism.
- Where possible, establishing mechanisms to allow workers to provide services from home if public health officials advise against non-essential travel outside the home.
- Establishing partnerships with other members of the sector to provide mutual support and maintenance of essential services during a pandemic.

Individuals and Families

The critical role of individuals and families in controlling a pandemic cannot be overstated. Modeling of the transmission of influenza vividly illustrates the impact of one individual's behavior on the spread of disease, by showing that an infection carried by one person can be transmitted to tens or hundreds of others. For this reason, individual action is perhaps the most important element of pandemic preparedness and response.

Education on pandemic preparedness for the population should begin before a pandemic, should be provided by all levels of government and the private sector, and should occur in the context of preventing the transmission of any infection, such as the annual influenza or the common cold. Responsibilities of the individual and families include:

- Taking precautions to prevent the spread of infection to others if an individual or a family member has symptoms of influenza.
- Being prepared to follow public health guidance that may include limitation of attendance at public gatherings and nonessential travel for several days or weeks.

- Keeping supplies of materials at home, as recommended by authorities, to support essential needs of the household for several days if necessary.

International Partners

We rely upon our international partnerships, with the United Nations, international organizations and private non-profit organizations, to amplify our efforts, and will engage them on a multilateral and bilateral basis. Our international effort to contain and mitigate the effects of an outbreak of pandemic influenza is a central component of our overall strategy. In many ways, the character and quality of the U.S. response and that of our international partners may play a determining role in the severity of a pandemic.

The International Partnership on Avian and Pandemic Influenza stands in support of multinational organizations. Members of the Partnership have agreed that the following 10 principles will guide their efforts:

1. International cooperation to protect the lives and health of our people;
2. Timely and sustained high-level global political leadership to combat avian and pandemic influenza;
3. Transparency in reporting of influenza cases in humans and in animals caused by virus strains that have pandemic potential, to increase understanding and preparedness and especially to ensure rapid and timely response to potential outbreaks;
4. Immediate sharing of epidemiological data and samples with the World Health Organization (WHO) and the international community to detect and characterize the nature and evolution of any outbreaks as quickly as possible, by utilizing, where appropriate, existing networks and mechanisms;
5. Rapid reaction to address the first signs of accelerated transmission of H5N1 and other highly pathogenic influenza strains so that appropriate international and national resources can be brought to bear;
6. Prevent and contain an incipient epidemic through capacity building and in-country collaboration with international partners;
7. Work in a manner complementary to and supportive of expanded cooperation with and appropriate support of key multilateral

organizations (including the WHO, Food and Agriculture Organization and World Organization for Animal Health);

8. Timely coordination of bilateral and multilateral resource allocations; dedication of domestic resources (human and financial); improvements in public awareness; and development of economic and trade contingency plans;
9. Increased coordination and harmonization of preparedness, prevention, response and containment activities among nations, complementing domestic and regional preparedness initiatives, and encouraging where appropriate the development of strategic regional initiatives; and
10. Actions based on the best available science.

Through the Partnership and other bilateral and multilateral initiatives, we will promote these principles and support the development of an international capacity to prepare, detect and respond to an influenza pandemic.

INDEX

A

B

C

D

E

F

G

H

S

T

U

V

W

Y